The Curti Lectures

The University of Wisconsin–Madison
September 1978

To honor the distinguished historian Merle Curti,
lectures in social and intellectual history
were inaugurated in 1976 under the sponsorship of the
University of Wisconsin Foundation and the
Department of History of the University of Wisconsin–Madison.

Published by the University of Wisconsin Press

Christopher Hill, *Some Intellectual Consequences of the English Revolution* (1980)

Fighting the Plague in Seventeenth-Century Italy

Carlo M. Cipolla

THE UNIVERSITY OF WISCONSIN PRESS

Published 1981

The University of Wisconsin Press
114 North Murray Street
Madison, Wisconsin 53715

The University of Wisconsin Press, Ltd.
1 Gower Street
London WC1E 6HA, England

First printing

Printed in the United States of America

For LC CIP information see the colophon

ISBN 0-299-08340-3 cloth; 08344-6 paper

Contents

v

Tables

Figures

Preface

The three chapters of this book comprise the Curti Lectures which I had the honor of delivering at the University of Wisconsin–Madison in September 1978. I take this opportunity to express my gratitude to the Department of History at the University of Wisconsin–Madison for the invitation to give the lectures and to all those who entertained me at Madison on the occasion.

The research on which the book is based was largely supported by the National Institutes of Health, Research Grant no LM02324 from the National Library of Medicine.

In the preparation of the text I was privileged in receiving advice and help from a number of scholars and friends. I should like to mention especially G. Brieger, E. Cecchi, E. Coturri, L. Del Panta, G. Doria, N. Howard-Jones, M. Kittel, J. Schachter, and M. Spallanzani.

The Institute of International Studies at the University of California, Berkeley, assisted me financially and otherwise both in the research as well as in the preparation of the manuscript. The staff of the Institute has been extremely generous both with time and patience in dealing with my persistent requests.

It is a pleasure for me to thank here all those individuals and institutions that in one way or another have helped me in my work.

Fighting the Plague
in Seventeenth-Century Italy

Abbreviations

used in the footnotes for reference to documents

ASF: Archivio di Stato di Firenze
ASP: Archivio di Stato di Pistoia

Note

All the Tuscan documents referred to in this book carry dates in the Florentine calendar. In contrast to the modern calendar, the Florentine year began on March 25. Thus a Florentine waking up on the morning of January 1 would not think of living in a new year, and in dating documents he would not change the year. He would do so only on and after March 25.

In the following pages all dates have been changed from Florentine to modern notation.

Introduction

After the great pandemic of 1348 the plague became endemic in Europe, and for more than three centuries epidemics of plague kept flaring up in one area after another. The recurrent outbreaks of the disease deeply affected European life at all levels—the demographic as well as the economic, the social as well as the political, the artistic as well as the religious.

To state that the plague is the villain in the stories that follow is an oversimplified abstraction. The real villains are the microbe known today under the name of *Yersinia pestis*, the rats which harbored the microbe, the fleas that carried the microbe from infected rats to men, and the widespread poverty and filth which favored the proliferation of both rats and fleas in human dwellings. For the moment, however, let us ignore such details and let us assume that the villain is the plague.

For a better understanding of the stories that follow, it is necessary to have some precise notions about the nature, characteristics, and behavior of the plague in the period under scrutiny. The interested reader will find the information in Appendix A. Here I want to stress that the book is not devoted to the villain. It is devoted instead to the desperate battle that a handful of dedicated men fought against a most dreaded, invisible enemy under impossible conditions.

In order to fight the plague, the major states of Northern Italy had developed a system of public health. The first rudimentary steps were taken at the time of the pandemic of 1348, and by the middle of the sixteenth century the system had reached a high degree of complexity and sophistication. The system was based on special Magistracies which combined legislative, judicial, and executive powers (hence the title of Magistracies) in all matters pertaining to public health. As I have shown elsewhere,[1] in the course of time the Health Magistrates progressively expanded the sphere of their controls to such matters as the recording of deaths, burials, the marketing of food, the sewage system, the disposal of byproducts of various economic activities, the hospitals, the hostelries, prostitution, and so on. The widening scope of their authority and action, however, did not imply any shift of emphasis in their main interest and preoccupation. Their main purpose remained the prevention and control of epidemics; their constant nightmare remained the plague.

By the middle of the sixteenth century all the major cities of Northern Italy had permanent Magistracies of public health; the minor cities and the rural communities set up health boards only in time of emergency. Both the permanent boards of the major cities and the temporary boards of the minor communities were subordinate and directly answerable to the central Health Magistracies of their respective capitals.[2]

Following the Italian example, similar developments took place north of the Alps, but health organizations outside of Italy remained at a more primitive level throughout the sixteenth and seventeenth centuries. Within the Italian peninsula itself, south of Florence developments were late and the health organization remained relatively rudimentary. As late as 1613 it was recorded that ''in Siena there is no Magistracy for Public Health; the Balìa[3] is the supreme Magistracy''; and members of the Balìa were asked to serve as Deputies for public health when the necessity arose.[4] In 1628 the Florentine Ambassador reported that

1. See Cipolla, *Public Health and the Medical Profession*, Chap. 1.
2. In Tuscany, however, the Health Magistracy of the free port of Leghorn claimed autonomy from the central Supreme Health Magistracy of Florence; see below, Chap. 2, fn. 6.
3. The *Balìa* was the highest administrative body in Siena.
4. ASF, Sanità, Negozi, b. 136, c. 1259 (23 October 1613).

in Rome "there are no officers for Public Health; the Conservators of Rome, that is, the main Magistracy of the City, appoint officers for Public Health only when there is suspicion of an epidemic."[5] In Naples there was a relatively undeveloped structure, typically characterized by corruption and inefficiency, as shown in the episode mentioned in Chapter 2.

Thus the region centered around the cities of Venice, Milan, Genoa, and Florence was by far the most developed area in Europe in regard to health organization. The organizational genius was not, however, matched by medical knowledge, and the efficacy of the ideas, institutions, and legislation developed in Northern Italy in matters of public health suffered badly from the medical ignorance of the period. The Health Magistrates did their best to fight the recurrent epidemics of plague, but what constituted the plague they did not know: they were provided with totally absurd notions concerning the etiology of the disease and the mechanism of its propagation. As I wrote elsewhere,[6] their preventive measures were no more than shots in the dark. People were groping blindly when fighting the plague, as we are now when fighting neoplasms. And working in the dark leads to errors, wasted resources, and accusations against innocents. Some of the measures taken were actually counterproductive; others were unnecessarily severe. On the other hand, repeated observation suggested some valid ideas which gave rise to ordinances, the wisdom of which no one would now think of questioning. I shall return to this point in Chapter 1. Here it is important to stress that the health ordinances were at best sources of great annoyance and severe privation and thus met with strong opposition. The segregation of entire families, the separation of kindred in the horror of pesthouses, the closing of markets and trade, the consequent rise of unemployment, the

5. ASF, Sanità, Negozi, b. 142, c. 888 (26 February 1628).
6. Cipolla, *Public Health and the Medical Profession*, Chap. 1, and Cipolla, *Faith, Reason, and the Plague*, Chap. 2.

burning of furnishings and goods, the prohibition of religious assemblies, the requisitioning of monasteries for use as hospitals— all these and similar measures provoked reactions which often acquired violent tones. Life was not easy for the health officers of the time. They fought a desperate battle against a formidable and yet invisible enemy. Paradoxically, their action made them highly unpopular among the people whom they were trying to protect. By focusing attention on specific episodes, the essays collected in this volume are intended to show the many fronts on which the health officers had to fight their battle and the many odds that were against them.

CHAPTER 1

Theory, Observation, and Policy

When a severe epidemic of influenza afflicted Sicily in 1557 and 1558, Dr. G. F. Ingrassia, while addressing the administration of Palermo, made a statement that in fact was an admonition: "Your Lordships do not seek from us physicians information about our therapies because it is our responsiblity to deliver them to the individual patients; what Your Lordships seek from us is advice on how to provide for the collectivity.'"[1] In other words, therapy should be solely the concern of the physician who was directly responsible to the patient; the health boards should "provide for the collectivity" in terms of prevention.

The fields of competence, however, were not and could not be so neatly separated. Doctors concerned themselves not only with therapy but with prevention as well, and they were supposed to provide the health boards with technical advice on both aspects. Moreover, because current therapies so often proved to be of no value against the plague, the doctors themselves were inclined to put more emphasis on prevention than on therapy. During the plague epidemic of 1576 the Genoese physician Giovan Agostino Contardo wrote a small treatise on "How to preserve and cure oneself of the plague"; in it he remarked that in medicine "prevention is much more noble and more necessary than therapy.'"[2]

1. Ingrassia, *Ragionamento*, quoted by Giuffre, "L'epidemia d'influenza," p. 7.
2. Contardo, *Il modo di preservarsi*, p. 5.

Such concepts have a remarkable air of modernity. Unfortunately, their application was misdirected and muddled by the prevalence of incorrect ideas about the etiology of infectious disease. With regard to the plague, the basic, predominant idea was that it originated from venomous atoms. Whether generated by rotting matter or emanating from infected persons, animals, or objects, the venomous atoms would infect salubrious air and make it "miasmatic"—that is, poisonous. It was indeed the "corruption" of the air that, according to the doctors of the Renaissance, was the basic precondition for the outbreak of an epidemic of plague.

Besides being deadly poisonous, the nasty atoms were also exceptionally "sticky": they would "stick" to inanimate objects, animals, and human beings in the same way that perfumes and foul odors permeate fabrics and other materials. When inhaled or absorbed through the pores of the skin by a person or by an animal, the venomous atoms would poison the body, cause infirmity and, owing to their extreme malignity, in most cases would bring death. By direct contact or by inhalation the atoms could actually pass from one object to another, from one person to the next, from one object or an animal to a person and vice versa. It logically followed that the only way to avoid the spreading of the disease was to stop all intercourse with people, animals, and objects coming from areas afflicted by the plague.

Despite nebulous phraseology, the basic theory was simple, logical, and internally consistent. But simplicity, logicality, and consistency were not and never are assurances of validity. In fact the theoretical system in question hardly amounted to more than dogmatic ignorance. We should not laugh, however, at the doctors of the Renaissance: even today, three centuries after the Scientific Revolution, an alarming number of self-styled social scientists seem to believe that if their models are logical and consistent they ought to be accurate. This is obviously not the case.

The real test of accuracy is observation—unquestionably so, with some important provisos.

Man cannot grasp new facts without reference to some existing concepts, and these concepts inevitably modify the kinds of facts he sees and how he sees them. When an investigator observes reality, he does not operate in a vacuum. He is of his own age and society. The very words and concepts that he uses have peculiar connotations which are determined by time and space and which in turn condition his thoughts and reasoning. He is never immune from a more or less consciously presumed conceptual system of reference. The most induction-addicted investigator never starts from a *tabula rasa*.

Actually, if the prevalent paradigm is totally alien to the reality under scrutiny the investigator may not even notice what passes before his eyes (as the history of the microscope in its first centuries of existence testifies); if the investigator does take notice of the phenomenon, he may be induced to discard it as irrelevant. The fact of the matter is that what one observes is only an infinitesimal particle of reality; and that particle acquires a meaning only if it fits into a related mosaic. If the right mosaic is not there, if there is nothing to which the minute tile can be related, the tile looks insignificant and carries no message. Only the exceptional genius can conceive the whole universe from a glance at a little particle. If all this sounds preposterously abstract, let me quote a telling episode which is relevant to the subject of this book.

Early in the seventeenth century, the doctors in France who visited patients suffering from the plague started to wear a robe made of *toile-cirée,* that is fine linen cloth coated with a paste made of wax mixed with some aromatic substances.[3] The sinister

---

3. On the origin and the characteristics of the costume see Salzmann, "Masques portés par les médecins," pp. 5–14.

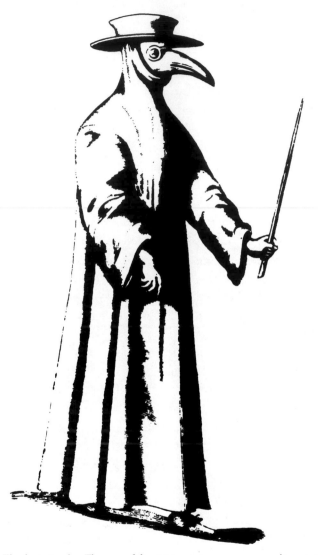

Figure 1. The doctor's robe. The nose of the sinister costume was supposed to act as a filter, being filled with materials imbued with perfumes and alleged disinfectants. The lenses were also supposed to protect the eyes from the miasmas. Illustration from *Historiarum anatomicarum medicarum rariorum* (1661), by Thomas Bartholin.

costume (Fig. 1) became very popular, especially in Italy,[1] and during the epidemic of 1630–31 it was commonly used not only in large cities such as Bologna,[5] Lucca,[6] and Florence,[7] but also in minor Tuscan communities such as Montecarlo, Pescia, and Poppi.[8] When another epidemic of plague ravaged parts of Italy

4. P. Furst in Germany in 1656 and Dr. Manger in Geneva in 1721 described the wax robe as an Italian medical costume, ignoring its French origin.

5. Brighetti, *Bologna e la peste*, p. 69.

6. In his report on the plague of 1630 in Verona, Dr. Pona recorded that "During this bad epidemic, following the practice of the French physicians, the town of Lucca made a provision that the plague-doctors ought to wear a long robe of thin, waxed cloth. The robe had to be hooded and the doctors had to visit the patients with the head covered and wearing spectacles" (*Il gran contagio*, p. 30).

7. According to an anonymous but well-informed writer, during the epidemic of 1630–31 in Florence, "physicians, surgeons, and apothecaries wore a robe made of waxed cloth and garnished with a red color; this sort of apparel is useful and protects from contagion and for this reason is also worn by the clergymen when they administer the sacraments to the sick" (Catellacci, ed., "Curiosi ricordi," p. 38. See also Rondinelli, *Relazione del contagio*, p. 54). The stretches used to carry the patients to the pesthouses were also covered with waxed cloth (Catellacci, p. 384).

A curious notation in a letter by Cardinal Giovan Carlo de' Medici seems to suggest that the robe used in Florence covered the person only to his knees (see Bini, "La peste," p. 273, n. 55).

8. By 1630 the technique of producing the waxed robe had not yet spread to the minor centers of Tuscany, but doctors and clergymen alike knew of the existence of the robe and often requested it. On June 1, 1631, the administration of Pescia informed the health board of Florence that a master Nicolò Biagi from Lucca had accepted to serve as community surgeon during the epidemic but he requested, among other things, to be provided with "a waxed robe of the kind that the surgeons of Florence wear" (ASF, Sanità, Negozi, b. 158, c. 11). On June 13, 1631, the Community of Montecarlo requested from the health board in Florence "a waxed robe for the surgeon because here there is no person who knows how to wax a robe as it is done in Florence" (ibid., c. 482). On August 16, 1631, the health board of Florence despatched two waxed robes to two friars who served in the pesthouse at Poppi (ASF, Sanità, Partiti, b. 9, c. 9v).

Curiously enough, in 1630 the waxed robe was seemingly unknown in Piedmont despite the close relationships of this region with France. A Piedmontese ordinance of 1630 established that physicians, surgeons, and barbers had to wear clothing made of silk "or other material with little or no hair" (Borelli, *Editti antichi*, p. 659, cap. 17).

in 1656–57, the costume was again commonly used in Rome[9] and in Genoa.[10] The idea behind the making and the adoption of the waxed robe was that the venomous atoms of the miasmas would not "stick" to its smooth and slippery surface. Because its use seemingly worked and served its purpose, the doctors of the time found in that fact a confirmation of their theories about contagion and the role of miasmas.

Father Antero Maria da San Bonaventura was a bright and energetic friar who was charged with the administration of the main pesthouse at Genoa during the epidemic of 1657. Experience taught him that those who went to serve in the pesthouse and who had not been previously infected with the plague rarely failed to contract the disease. He had no faith in the precautions currently practiced, and about the robe made from waxed cloth, this is what he had to say: "The waxed robe in a pesthouse is good only to protect one from the fleas which cannot nest in it.'"[11] The observation by the friar about the waxed robe was both accurate and perceptive: the robe did not protect people from the miasmas, it protected people from the fleas.[12]

9. In Rome during the epidemic of 1656 the plague doctors not only had to wear the waxed robe but they also had to have their carriages covered with a waxed cloth. See Savio, "Ricerche sulla peste," p. 117.

While reporting a curious anecdote about Dr. Giovanni Prescia, Cardinal Gastaldi writes that when visiting the infected in the pesthouse the physician "had someone carrying in front of him a burning candle and a vase full of vinegar. Before taking the pulse he would immerse his hands in the vinegar. He also wore a robe of cloth made from flax which was completely waxed" (Gastaldi, *Tractatus*, pp. 69–71).

10. Antero, *Li lazaretti*, p. 518.

11. Ibid. See also p. 27.

12. To understand the origin of the remark by Father Antero, one has to go back to another passage in his book which describes the torment inflicted upon him by the hordes of fleas that infested the pesthouse: "I have to change my clothes frequently if I do not want to be devoured by the fleas, armies of which nest in my gown, nor have I force enough to resist them, and I need great strength of mind to keep still at the altar. If I want to rest for an hour in bed, I have to use a sheet, otherwise the lice would feast on my flesh; they vie with the fleas—the latter suck, the former bite. Someone may remark 'Oh, what nonsense

With this remark the friar had come incredibly close to an exceptional discovery. But he failed. In the prevailing system of thought the fleas were obnoxious but innocent animals. It followed that if the robe served only to protect people from the fleas it was useless against the plague. How could the friar possibly think of challenging the whole system on the basis of a casual remark about fleas? The theoretical system was universal and imposing. The observation about the fleas was incidental, almost humorous, and looked trivial even to its author. Thus the system prevailed and the observation was lost.

In the course of human experience thousands of brilliant and accurate observations must have gone astray simply because the related pieces of the mosaic were not there. Thousands of other observations suffered no less sad a destiny. Accurate observations may be manipulated to fit into a faulty conceptual system with the perverse result of lending support to it. The examples that one could quote are innumerable and would cover the past as well as the present, the sciences as well as the humanities, religion and philosophy as well as politics. Here I shall limit myself to the field and the time which are the subject of this book.

The people of the Renaissance did not fail to observe that in times of an epidemic persons who handled certain materials were more prone to catch the disease than persons who handled different materials. They recognized the dangerous nature of wool and woolens, cotton, hemp, flax, carpets, bags of grain, and the like. The observation was correct. Materials such as those just mentioned could easily harbor infected fleas. People did not, however, think in terms of microbes and their vectors, nor did they suspect the role of fleas. As indicated above, in relation to

---

you are saying.' Reader take pity on me, in the greatest of my sufferings. I can swear to you that all the bodily torments which are of necessity suffered in the lazaretti cannot compare even to the fleas, for they do not leave me even in the coldest depths of winter" (p. 176).

the story of the waxed robe, the doctors rationalized that the venomous atoms of the miasmas would "stick" more easily to hairy and rough surfaces than to smooth and hairless ones, in the same way that perfumes and foul odors would more easily saturate a piece of cloth than a piece of marble.

The people of the Renaissance also correctly recognized that the plague generally prevailed in the summer months. They failed to link the phenomenon with the life cycle of rats and fleas, but they had no difficulty reconciling it with their epidemiological theory: it was during the hottest months of the year that they smelled the foulest odors from the dirty streets, the faulty sewers, the sinks, the dung in the stables. Thus they correlated these facts and in the correlation found the "proof" that clearly the venomous miasmas grew out of rotting materials in the hot and humid climate of the summer. In this case as in the previous one, a corret observation served the unfortunate purpose of strengthening a false theory.

Paradoxical as it may sound, the lesson of history is that all too often people find it easier to manipulate the facts to fit their theories than to adapt their theories to the facts observed. When this happens the net result is a curious mixture of nonsense combined with sensible perceptions—which is indeed the description that one can give of the epidemiological theory that prevailed at the time of the Renaissance and during the Scientific Revolution in Western Europe.

To the pastiche of error and accuracy that prevailed at the theoretical level, there understandably corresponded a curious combination of nonsensensical provisions and enlightened measures at the policy level. The correspondence, however, was not absolute. Although the theoretical error generally produced nonsensical provisions and accurate observation produced some sensible measures, it also could happen that, when tempered at the practical level by common sense, theoretical error could originate sound action.

Let me quote an example. As previously mentioned, according to the prevailing medical theories an epidemic of plague originated from the corruption of the air, which in turn was caused by the venomous vapors emanating from rotting matter and filth. A common-sense sequitur to this view was that to avoid an outbreak or the further spread of an epidemic, the first and most important thing to do was to clean up the environment. Two centuries later, when cholera ravaged Europe, the English champions of the public health movement thought along exactly the same lines.

In Florence in 1630, Rondinelli reported that "after the disease had reached the neighboring towns of Parma, Piacenza, and Bologna," because of the growing and approaching danger, the Health Magistracy subdivided the city into six zones (*sestieri*)[13] and put each one of them under the supervision of gentlemen chosen from among the members of the Compagnia di San Michele, a lay religious society devoted to charitable pursuits. The gentlemen in question were asked "to visit the homes of the poor and have them thoroughly cleaned and repainted in order to get rid of anything that would produce foul odors because filth is the mother of the corruption of the air and the latter is the mother of the plague."[14]

That was not all. The Magistracy feared that in the houses of the lower orders people might sleep on old and filthy palliasses and, worrying about the harmful effects of filth, it instructed the gentlemen of the Compagnia to be alert to the problem and "to provide the poor with new palliasses or to have the straw of the palliasses changed whenever necessary." The situation turned out to be much worse than the Magistracy had suspected; indeed, the gentlemen of the Compagnia discovered a degree and diffusion of poverty absolutely unimaginable. So alarmed did they become that they did not wait to have the whole city

13. On the *sestieri*, see Rondinelli, *Relazione del contagio*, pp. 72 ff.
14. Ibid., p. 24.

surveyed, and in the early days of August 1630 the Compagnia hastened to forward to the Magistracy an interim report. It stated that the task force employed was made up of forty-eight gentlemen who so far had surveyed one-third of the city. The gentlemen had found only "very few sick people, hardly more than a dozen," but they had discovered that "in many houses there are no beds and people sleep on scattered straw and some have palliasses which are filthy and fetid." On the basis of this preliminary report the Magistracy immediately requested the Grand Duke to have some one thousand new palliasses ready for distribution among the poor, marked in such a way that they could neither be sold nor seized in payment of debts.[15] Less than a month later the Magistracy was in a position to determine exactly the number of new palliasses needed for each one of the six *sestieri* of the city:[16]

Sesto di San Giovanni	638
Sesto di Santa Maria Novella	148
Sesto di San Ambrogio	84
Sesto di Santa Croce	109
Sesto di Santo Spirito	225
Sesto di San Giorgio	143

Thus a total of 1347 new palliasses were distributed gratuitously among the poor in a city that counted less than twenty thousand families.

The burning of mattresses on which persons suffering from the plague had slept or died and their replacement by new mattresses was a measure normally resorted to in times of epidemics, but the operation carried out in Florence at the onset of the epidemic of 1630 was unique in the sense that the palliasses burned and substituted had belonged to healthy people. It was a truly preventive measure, born out of a totally erroneous theory and

15. ASF, Sanità, Rescritti, b. 37, c. 172 (12 August 1630).
16. ASF, Sanità, Negozi, b. 150, c. 53 (September 1630).

yet admirably sound even by modern standards, since old and filthy palliasses were a most likely receptacle of fleas.

Other instances of sound action born out of erroneous theory would not be difficult to list. suffice it to quote the distribution of waxed robes among doctors and confessors and the prompt isolation of infected individuals and their contacts. More often than not, however, erroneous theory misdirected efforts; when that was the case, good will and determination only served to waste both energies and resources.

As mentioned above, doctors thought that human intercourse was primarily responsible for the propagation of the plague. Thus when an epidemic broke out, most trade and communication were forbidden. Moreover, when the epidemic gave sign of subsiding, it was customary for the health authorities to decree a ''general quarantine,'' in the delusion of giving the final coup to the scourge. A ''general quarantine'' meant that as many people as possible had to remain locked up in their homes for a period of forty days, thus reducing to a minimum all human intercourse. When the ''general quarantine'' was decreed in Florence in the winter of 1630, the orders were that all females and males thirteen years of age and younger had to be quarantined in their homes. Owing to the efficiency of the Tuscan administration of the time, we can take a look at the costs involved in such operations. A survey was made and it was found that in a city of some 80,000 inhabitants, there were some 12,000 who normally would have been in need of some charity, however, under the condition of virtual blockade in which the city had been placed since the beginning of the epidemic, the number of the needy had increased to some 30,000.[17] In modern terms, the blockade of the city decreed in the name of health interests had caused unemployment to rise by some 150 percent. To feed a mass of

17. ASF, Sanità, Rescritti, b. 37, c. 665 (2 December 1630). See also Catellacci, ed., "Curiosi ricordi," p. 388, and Appendix A in this volume.

approximately 30,000 people quarantined for forty days, an additional organizational effort had to be mounted on the occasion of the general quarantine. Specifically, the administration employed in the operation 1,070 people, 23 mules, and 186 carriages with a total expenditure of 150,000 scudi.[18] And the sad fact is that all that effort was worse than useless; it was actually counterproductive because, as modern epidemiologists would point out, confining people where the source of infection was harbored meant increasing the risk of that infection.

All this sounds absurd, but fundamentally things have not changed. In our own days a noted physician pointedly remarked that he could not "think of any important human disease for which medicine possesses the outright capacity to prevent or cure where the cost of the technology is itself a major problem. . . . It is when physicians are bogged down by their incomplete technologies, by the innumerable things they are obliged to do in medicine when they lack a clear understanding of disease mechanisms, that the deficiencies of the health-care system are most conspicuous."[19] In other words, today as in the sixteenth and seventeenth centuries, costs are out of proportion to benefits when people are shooting in the dark.

The physicians and the health officers of those days fought against an enemy that they had not identified and whose mode of action they did not comprehend. In their impossible battle they were guided by some correct observations, but they were also misdirected by erroneous theories. Thus they were bogged down by the innumerable things that in their ignorance they felt that they had to do while they did not do the few things that they should have done. Under such conditions determination and good will largely served to expand the gap between costs and benefits.

18. Rondinelli, *Relazione del contagio*, pp. 71–72.
19. Lewis, *Lives of a Cell*, pp. 35–36.

Chapter 2

Public Health and International Relations

On June 14, 1652, the Genoese Health Magistracy notified its counterparts in Florence and other Northern Italian cities that "information has been received here in Genoa by qualified persons that in the city of Alghero in Sardinia contagious diseases have been uncovered which have caused the death of several people," and that consequently the Magistracy had proceeded to banish the city of Alghero and to suspend the entire island of Sardinia (Fig. 2).[1] As was customary in such cases, the printed proclamation of the ban and the suspension was enclosed with the message.

"Banishment" and "suspension" were technical terms commonly used to denote the interruption of regular trade and communication. No person, boat, merchandise, or letter from a banished or suspended area could enter the territory of the banishing state except at a few well-specified ports or places of entrance, where quarantine stations were set up. At the stations, incoming people, boats, and merchandise were subject to quarantine and disinfection even if they carried health certificates issued at the point of departure. In cases of exceptional danger the authorities reserved the right to refuse to admit people, boats, and merchandise from the banished areas even to the quarantine stations. People violating either the ban or the suspension, whether trying surreptitiously to enter the territory of the banishing state or sur-

1. ASF, Sanità, Negozi, b. 187, c. 96 (14 June 1652).

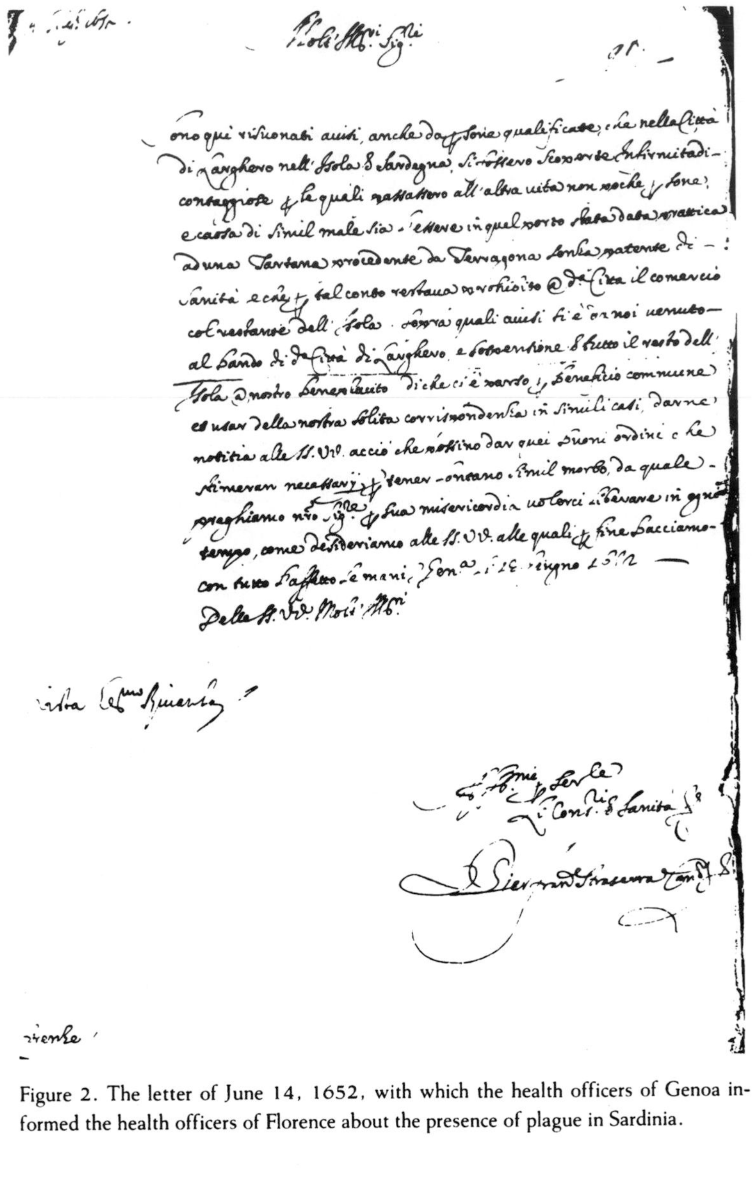
Molto Ill.ri Sig.ri

Sono qui risuonati avisi, anche da persone qualificate, che nella Città
di Langhero nell'Isola di Sardegna si scoprissero sospette Infirmitadi
contaggiose per le quali passassero all'altra vita non poche persone;
e causa di simil male sia stato in quel porto stata data prattica
a una Tartana procedente da Terragona senza patente di
Sanità e che per tal conto restava prohibito da detta Città il comercio
col restante dell'Isola. Sopra quali avisi si è da noi venuto
al Bando di detta Città di Langhero, e sospensione di tutto il resto dell'
Isola a nostro beneplacito di che ci è parso per beneficio commune
et usar della nostra solita corrispondenza in simili casi, darne
notitia alle SS. VV. acciò che possino dar quei buoni ordini che
stimeran necessarij per tener lontano simil morbo, da quale
preghiamo nostro Sig.re per sua misericordia volerci liberare in ogni
tempo, come desideriamo alle SS. VV. alle quali per fine bacciamo
con tutto l'affetto le mani. Gen.a 14 Giugno 1652

Delle SS. VV. Molto Ill.ri

Figure 2. The letter of June 14, 1652, with which the health officers of Genoa informed the health officers of Florence about the presence of plague in Sardinia.

reptitiously to introduce merchandise, were regarded as "bandits" and were therefore subject to capital punishment.

The difference between banishment and suspension was only a matter of degree. An area was banished when the presence of the plague had been "positively ascertained" and consequently it was understood that the ban would last for a long time and would not be repealed until some time after the end of the epidemic. Suspension, on the other hand, was adopted as a precautionary measure when the presence of the plague had not been "ascertained" but when there was a legitimate suspicion that the area could become infected either because of proximity and frequent intercourse with a banished area, or because of laxity in the enforcement of health controls, or both.[2] Being based not on fact but merely on presumption, a suspension was decreed "*a beneplacito,*" that is, it could be repealed as easily and promptly as it had been decreed. Moreover, a suspension would normally last only for a short period because it was soon changed into a ban if the "suspicion" proved correct, or it was repealed if the "suspicion" proved unfounded.

The notification issued by Genoa on June 14, 1652, was anything but exceptional. In the course of the sixteenth and seventeenth centuries the Health Magistracies of the capital cities of the republics and principalities of Northern Italy had firmly established the eminently civilized custom of regularly informing each other of all news that they gathered on health conditions prevailing in various parts of Italy, the rest of Europe, North Africa, and the Middle East. Florence "corresponded" regularly with Genoa, Venice, Verona, Milan, Mantua, Parma, Modena, Ferrara, Bologna, Ancona, and Lucca. The frequency of the correspondence with each one of these places ranged from one letter every two weeks in periods of calm to several messages a week in times of emergency.

2. ASF, Sanità, Negozi, b. 144, c. 249 (9 August 1629), c. 389 (7 September 1629).

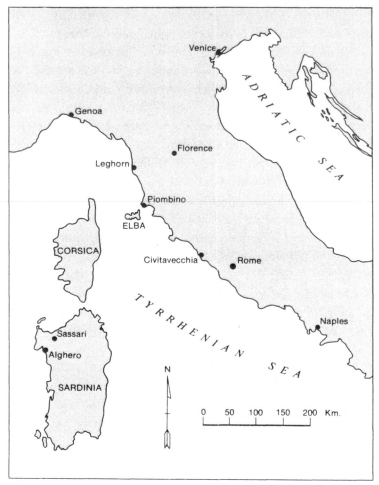

Figure 3. Northern and central Italy, with the islands of Corsica, Sardinia, and Elba.

What was exceptional in the Genoese message of June 14 was the gravity of the information. For months the Italian health authorities had been watching with trepidation the progress of the plague in the Mediterranean basin. The dread disease had been ravaging Catalonia in Spain and Languedoc in France. Then it had spread to Majorca. Now, as Genoa reported, it had appeared in Sardinia.

The island of Sardinia is some two hundred miles away from the Tuscan coast, and there was an intense traffic to and from the island. Memories of the havoc caused by the epidemic of 1630 were still fresh in most people's minds and served only to create a more tense atmosphere.

On June 19 Genoa issued another alarming message. A Genoese vessel which had left Alghero ten days before had arrived in Genoa, and the captain reported that while in Alghero the scrivener of the boat had died, possibly of plague. The Health Magistracy of Genoa reassured its correspondents that the belongings of the scrivener had been publicly burned and that the boat with its crew and its cargo had been quarantined at the new pier away from the city under the guard of German mercenaries.[3]

The news from Genoa elicited immediate and alarmed reactions. On June 20, having received the message of June 14 but not yet the message of June 19, the Health Magistracy in Florence advised the Grand Duke of Tuscany to follow Genoa's steps. The Grand Duke gave his approval on the twenty-second, and on the twenty-fifth the ban on Alghero and the suspension of Sardinia were publicly proclaimed.[4] The neighboring Republic of Lucca and the city of Bologna had already taken the same measure on the eighteenth and the twenty-second, respectively.[5]

The Supreme Health Magistracy of the Grand Duchy of Tus-

3. ASF, Sanità, Negozi, b. 187, c. 102 (19 June 1652).
4. ASF, Sanità, Negozi, b. 187, c. 106 (20 June 1652), c. 109 (25 June 1652); ASF, Sanità, Partiti, b. 13, c. 13 (20 June 1652); Biblioteca, Bandi Sanità, vol. 2.
5. ASF, Sanità, Negozi, b. 187, c. 99 (18 June 1652), c. 105 (22 June 1652).

cany was seated in Florence. In Leghorn, the main Tuscan port, there was another major Health Magistracy, which always claimed to be answerable not to the Magistracy in Florence but solely and directly to the Grand Duke.⁶ In Pisa there was a health board which was answerable to the Magistracy in Florence, but in times of emergency it was authorized to take urgent measures on its own initiative—with the understanding that such measures had to be approved subsequently by the magistrates in Florence. When the news about the Sardinian developments reached Leghorn and Pisa, the local authorities entered a state of great agitation, which is perfectly understandable if one considers that both cities are situated on the coast and were more directly exposed than Florence to all dangers coming from the sea. On June 22 the Health Magistracy in Florence was informed that Leghorn and Pisa had taken urgent measures to increase vigilance along the coast in order to prevent the landing of all boats coming from Sardinia and Corsica.⁷

Up to this point nobody had mentioned Corsica. Corsica, however, is adjacent to Sardinia, and communication between the two islands was both frequent and intense. It is perfectly understandable that in consideration of both geographical and commercial factors the health authorities should look with apprehension at boats coming from Corsica, but no case of infection had been reported from the island and the orders to prevent the landing of boats from Corsica were therefore premature and questionable, to say the least. There was even more that was questionable. Corsica was a Genoese dominion. Decency and etiquette requested that before taking a drastic measure concern-

---

6. ASF, Sanità, Negozi, b. 189, c. 791 (5 December 1654): "Il Magistrato della Sanità di Livorno ha sempre preteso et pretende di non havere altro superiore che il Granduca." On the health board of Leghorn, see Ciano, *La Sanità Marittima*, which also contains references to the story described above.

7. ASF, Sanità, Negozi, b. 187, c. 104 (22 June 1652); ASF, Sanità, Partiti, b. 13, c. 14 (24 June 1652); ASF, Mediceo, b. 2327 (24 June 1652).

ing Corsican boats the Tuscan health authorities should have asked for information from Genoa or should at least have warned the Genoese of their intentions. Nothing of the kind was done. The Health Magistrates of Florence ratified unconditionally the action by the authorities in Leghorn and Pisa, and to their justification one can only say that possibly the magistrates acted under personal pressure from the Grand Duke.[8] But they must have felt uncomfortable. Only a few years earlier, in 1648, when during an epidemic of typhus Rome had banished Tuscany without previously consulting Florence, the Florentines had called the action "a mere caprice of bad will" done in violation of "the proper rules."[9] Now they had acted in the same manner.

The provisions regarding the Corsican boats were not publicized. The Florentine Magistracy mentioned them in a letter to Lucca on June 25 because it wanted the neighboring republic to adopt similar measures,[10] but in a letter written that very day to Genoa the Magistracy simply reported the adoption of measures "to prevent the landing of people proceeding from places which are infected or suspect," entirely failing to mention that now the Tuscans regarded Corsica as "suspect."[11]

The letter to Lucca must have been sent by special courier, and on June 26 Lucca hastened to inform Florence that it "intended to give the same secret orders" to her coastal guards.[12] "Secret orders," however, cannot be kept secret for long if they have to be enforced, and on June 27 the Health Magistracy in Florence—possibly again under the personal pressure of the Grand Duke—decided to formally banish the entire island of Sardinia and suspend the entire island of Corsica. The ordi-

8. ASF, Mediceo, b. 2327, Consulta of June 24; ASF, Sanità, Copialettere, b. 65, cc. 6v and 8v (25 June 1652).
9. ASF, Sanità, Negozi, b. 183, c. 471 (14 August 1648).
10. ASF, Sanità, Copialettere, b. 65, c. 6 (25 June 1652).
11. ASF, Sanità, Copialettere, b. 65, c. 9 (25 June 1652).
12. ASF, Sanità, Negozi, b. 187, c. 138 (26 June 1652).

nance was proclaimed on June 28, and at the express wish of the Grand Duke gallows were erected along the coast to demonstrate determination to enforce the law.[13]

The day after the proclamation, on June 29, the Florentine Magistracy hastened to send a copy of the new ordinance to its counterpart in Lucca,[14] but it hesitated to inform the Magistracy of Genoa, thus showing once more its embarrassment. In the meantime, on June 28 Genoa answered the Florentine letter of June 25 with a diplomatic message.[15] Florence had mentioned its orders preventing landings of boats ''proceeding from places which are infected or suspect,'' but had not explicitly mentioned Corsica. The Genoese Magistracy began its letter by praising the diligence of the Tuscans. It went on to convey information received from Barcelona regarding the progress of the plague in Catalonia. And it continued:

> We have also seen excerpts from a letter written by a person in Tuscany to his correspondent here with the information that Your Lordships have suspended two places in Corsica and others in Sardinia on suspicion of contagion. As far as Corsica is concerned there must have been a misunderstanding. If we had known of any case of contagion in Corsica we would have been negligent in not informing you, with the sincerity that we profess to everybody. Therefore we have not given any credit to the news, in consideration of the fact that every day boats arrive here from Corsica; yesterday a boat arrived which had left Ajaccio eight days earlier, and we learned that in that island people enjoy good health. Your Lordships must believe that if there had been any new development we would not have been the last to inform you.

A few days later the Genoese made a good show of their ''sincerity.'' A surgeon in the health service uncovered a case of plague on a boat from Sardinia that was anchored at the new pier

13. ASF, Sanità, Partiti, b. 13, c. 14v (27 June 1652); ASF, Sanità, Copialettere, b. 65, cc. 9–10 (27 June 1652); ASF, Sanità, Negozi, b. 187, cc. 142, 145 (28 June 1652); ASF, Mediceo, b. 2327 (28 June 1652).
14. ASF, Sanità, Copialettere, b. 65, c. 13 (29 June 1652).
15. ASF, Sanità, Negozi, b. 187, c. 146 (28 June 1652).

for purposes of the quarantine, and plague was also recognized at the pesthouse in a passenger from the same boat. The Genoese authority hastened to inform the Health Magistracies of Northern Italy, adding, of course, detailed and reassuring information concerning all the precautions that had been taken to prevent the spread of the infection. The letter sent to Florence with this information is dated July 1, 1652.[16] In the meantime the Florentines had received the Genoese note of June 28. They could no longer delay officially informing Genoa of their suspension of Corsica. This they did on July 2.[17] Their note was received in Genoa on July 5—and it created a furor. The Genoese answered immediately with a letter which, judging from the styles and the inks, must have been dictated and written at different times. In the heat of the discussion the Health Magistracy had clearly split into two factions. The moderate faction must have inspired the first part of the letter, in which the Genoese Magistracy limited itself to a passionate protest against the grossly undiplomatic behavior of the Tuscans. The other faction, however, managed to prevail (though by a slim majority),[18] and it carried the day with a resolution which is reported in the second half of the letter: Genoa suspended the Tuscan harbor of Piombino and the Tuscan islands of Elba and Pianosa.[19] This was clearly an act of retaliation, taken under the pretext that the Republic of Lucca had allegedly taken a similar measure—which was not true.[20]

Within the following three or four days Florence received messages in dramatic succession. First the Genoese letter of July 1 arrived, in which the Genoese gave notice of the two

16. ASF, Sanità, Negozi, b. 187, c. 175 (1 July 1652).
17. ASF, Sanità, Copialettere, b. 65, c. 13 (2 July 1652).
18. The information is contained in the report by an informer; see ASF, Mediceo, b. 2327 (20 July 1652).
19. ASF, Sanità, Negozi, b. 187, c. 189 (5 July 1652).
20. Lucca protested having been used as an excuse by Genoa; see ASF, Sanità, Negozi, b. 187, c. 230.

cases of plague; then the other Genoese letter of July 5 arrived, which announced the suspension of Piombino, Elba, and Pianosa; then there arrived an urgent message dated July 7 from the Governor of Leghorn, who informed the Grand Duke that boats from Corsica prevented by the ordinance of June 28 from coming to Tuscany were circumventing the suspension by going first to Genoa, taking a Genoese patent, and then appearing in Leghorn as Genoese vessels.[21]

The Florentines did not need to be prodded. They were nervous because of the impending danger, and in addition they were suspicious of those clever and supercilious Genoese. The formal expressions of reciprocal consideration which are so abundant in the correspondence between the Florentine and Genoese authorities should not deceive us. The overall relationship between the Grand Duchy and the Republic was strained by economic rivalry: on the one hand, Genoa regarded the rapidly growing free port of Leghorn as a menace to her mercantile interests; on the other hand, the Tuscans were traditionally mistrustful of the Genoese and were obsessively fearful that those clever merchants were spending their days and nights plotting schemes to ruin the growing fortunes of Leghorn.[22] In Tuscany the Genoese were not very popular. A note from Florence to Leghorn referred not without resentment to the Genoese sailors as bullish characters "who pretend to land regardless of any rules,"[23] and a note written by a high-ranking officer from Leghorn to Florence referred to the Genoese as people "who preach rigor to others

21. ASF, Mediceo, b. 2327 (7 July 1652).

22. Such views were reflected also in the reports of the Venetian Resident in Florence to the Doge and the Venetian Senate. In his report of January 17, 1665, commenting on the lack of trade in Leghorn, the Venetian Resident wrote that "Genoa never loses an opportunity of making things worse" (*Calendar of State Papers*, Vol. 34, Venice, 1664–66 [London, 1933], p. 176, no. 20). On the rivalry between Leghorn and Genoa and its influence on the action of the health board, see Toniolo Fascione, "L'attività processuale," pp. 28 ff. See also Ciano, *La Sanità Marittima*.

23. ASF, Sanità, Copialettere, b. 65, cc. 9–10 (27 June 1652).

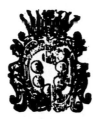

BANDO
PER CAVSA DI PESTE.

 L Sereniſſ. Gran Duca di Toſcana, e per S.A.S. Li SS. Vfiziali di Sanità della Città di Firenze; ſentito, che il mal contagioſo di Peſte fa progreſſi notabili, & opera effetti ſpauenteuoli nell'Iſola, e Regno di Sardigna; E ſtante gl'auuiſi, che danno ſi SS. Conſeruadori della Sanità di Genoua con lor lettere del primo Luglio di due caſi di Peſte ſeguiti ſopra vaſcelli, che di Sardigna ſon cóparſi in quantità in quel Porto, e quiui ammeſſi ſotto buone gnardie, per quanto ſcriuano i medeſimi SS. Conſeruatori : e ſtante il Bando, che veglia di tutta la Sardigna, donde non ſi ammettono nelli Stati di S. A. vaſcelli di ſorte alcuna prouenienti da detta Iſola, ma ſi ſcacciano aſſolutamente; Fanno per il preſente publico Bando ſoſpendere, e ſoſpendono il Commerzio per ſino à nuouo ordine, con la detta Città di Genoua, e ſuo Dominio, proibendo ad ogni perſona, che veniſſe, ò paſſaſſe da i luoghi del Genoueſato il potere entrare nelli Stati di S. A. ancorche per breue ſpazio, ò ſemplice paſſaggio, & anco il potere in eſſi introdurre robe, ò mercanzie di qualſiuoglia ſorte, che perueniſſero dalla detta Città di Genoua, e ſuo Dominio, ſotto pena della Vita, confiſcazione de beni, perdita delle robe, & animali, ancorche non fuſſero proprie del conduttore di quelle, applicate dette confiſcazioni, e perdita di robe per vn quarto al notificatore ſegreto, ò paleſe, & il reſtante al loro Vfizio; e nella medeſima pena incorreranno quelli, che deſſero ricetto in queſti Stati alle dette perſone, mercanzie, e robe, che fuſſero introdotte contro alla diſpoſizione del preſente Bando; e tutto à chiara à notizia di ciaſcuno, &c. Mandantes, &c.

Antonio Dei Cancell.

Bandito per me Lorenzo del Noia Banditore il di 10. di Luglio 1652.

_____

IN FIRENZE nella Stamperia di S. A. S 1652.

Figure 4. The order issued on July 10, 1652, by the Health Magistracy in Florence, suspending trade with Genoa.

29

while they resort to leniency whenever they think it is in their own interest.''[24]

On July 10, on the grounds that while no Sardinian boats were admitted to the harbors of the Grand Duchy, "numerous boats" continued to arrive in Genoa from Sardinia and two cases of plague had been identified, the Health Magistracy in Florence took the serious step of "suspending until further orders all trade with the City of Genoa and its dominions" (see Fig. 4).[25]

The news took Genoa by surprise, but the Genoese reacted without delay. They had heard that, some time earlier, two boats from Sardinia which had not been allowed to enter the harbor of Bastia in Corsica had been admitted to Leghorn. This was as good an excuse as any. On July 13 Genoa decreed the suspension of Leghorn.[26] The two powers were now openly at loggerheads.

What happened in those and the following days shows how interdependent had become the health services of Northern Italy and how sensitive was their network of information. On July 11, Florence hastened to inform Milan, Mantua, Parma, Modena, Ferrara, Bologna, Ancona, Lucca, Verona, and Venice of the suspension of Genoa. For its part Genoa informed all her correspondents first of the suspension of Piombino, Elba, and Pianosa, and later of the suspension of Leghorn. In turn, each of the recipients of the information hurriedly passed it on to the others, and everybody requested more information from the contenders. Florence bluntly asserted that the Genoese measure had been taken "ad vindictam" ("as a reprisal"). Messages crossed each other at a frantic pace, and each power had then to decide which steps to take on the basis of the contradictory information available. Lucca, Rome, Mantua, Ferrara, Bologna, and Venice

24. ASF, Mediceo, b. 2327 (13 September 1652).
25. ASF, Mediceo, b. 2327 (10 July 1652); and ASF, Biblioteca, Bandi Sanità, vol. 2.
26. ASF, Mediceo, b. 2327 (13 July 1652).

suspended Genoa and Corsica. Milan and Modena suspended Piombino, Elba, and Pianosa. The Prince of Massa and Carrara did not yield to Florentine pressure and refused to suspend Genoa and Corsica. In retaliation Florence suspended the principality." The whole business had reached the limits of absurdity. Even worse, the game between the two main contenders had reached a stalemate. The Grand Duke and his magistrates sensed that perhaps they had acted too precipitously. On the other hand, in Genoa there were people who thought that the Genoese reaction to the Tuscan move had not been the right one. But neither of the parties knew what to do next. As all too often happens in history, it had been much easier to start a conflict than to bring it to an end.

In the second half of July the Tuscan authorities were bothering their heads drafting a difficult letter to the Genoese Health Magistracy.[28] Pride prevented the Florentines from admitting that perhaps they had been wrong and that they wanted to resume normal relations with Genoa. They therefore sounded out the Genoese with an indirect approach. At the beginning of June a boat from Leghorn named *La Madonna della Speranza* had left Alexandria (Egypt). On her homeward journey, the boat had called at the harbor of Rosetta, where there had been an outbreak of plague. The captain, who disembarked, caught the infection. A few days later, after the boat had resumed its journey, the captain died, followed by the ship's surgeon and a sailor, both of whom had been attending the captain. When *La Madonna della Speranza* appeared at Leghorn she was denied admittance to the harbor.

Taking advantage of this tragic event, the Florentines dis-

27. ASF, Sanità, Negozi, b. 187, cc. 148, 180, 219, 251, 304, 308, 377, 383, 390, 425, 444, 486, 658; ASF, Mediceo, b. 2327 (16 July 1652).
28. ASF, Mediceo, b. 2327 (20 July 1652); ASF, Sanità, Partiti, b. 13, c. 22 (24 July 1652).

patched a special boat to Genoa to inform the Genoese of what had happened, just in case—they wrote in their message—the infected boat might try to call at the harbors of the Ligurian coast. The Florentine board took this occasion also to pass on the information that some Genoese passengers had appeared in Leghorn and that despite the suspension they had been allowed to disembark and move freely around after a pure formality of only three days' quarantine. Finally, the Florentines added, mail from Genoa was allowed to pass freely through Tuscany after it had been perfumed at the border stations. Neither the tone nor the substance of the message could have been more accommodating.

The answer of the Genoese Health Magistracy was polite in form but supercilious in substance. "We had already been informed of the arrival in Leghorn of that boat from Alexandria on which the Captain, the Surgeon, and a sailor had died of plague . . . and we also knew about the careful precautions taken in Leghorn." The obvious implications was that the Florentine communication was superfluous; the Genoese conceded, however, that the Florentines had sent their message "as a token of good correspondence for the sake of the common health," and as such they "were pleased to receive it." As to the fact that passengers from Genoa had been admitted to Leghorn after a quarantine of only three days despite the suspension, the Genoese were not at all ready to express appreciation; instead, they briskly commented: "We cannot help telling you that even that short quarantine was a superfluous precaution because, thanks be to God, in this City of Genoa as well as in Corsica people never enjoyed such good health as they presently enjoy, as Your Lordships can ascertain."[29]

The Genoese answer is dated July 25. It was brought back to Tuscany by the same boat which had been specially dispatched to Genoa. It arrived in Leghorn on July 28 and was read at the

29. ASF, Mediceo, b. 2327 (25 July 1652).

meeting of the Florentine Magistracy of July 29. The magistrates, who had been anxiously waiting for the Genoese answer, were more than ready to settle the dispute. Officially at least they did not take notice of the censorious posture of the Genoese, and on the basis of the reassurances provided by the Genoese in their letter, they recommended to the Grand Duke the lifting of the suspension of Genoa.[30] But the story was not destined to end there.

Grand Duke Ferdinand did not approve the recommendation of his Health Magistrates. He had other ideas, of which the magistrates were informed on July 30.[31] Since the Genoese had declared in their letter of June 25 that the city was in good health, "as your Lordships can ascertain," the Florentine court thought that it could use that phrase as an invitation to send to Genoa a mission of inquiry. The practice was not uncommon in seventeenth-century Italy. In earlier times an Italian state would rely on reports of secret informers. This custom had not been abandoned, but since the end of the sixteenth century it was complemented with the more civilized practice of official missions.[32] Typically a mission consisted of one medical person, either a physician or a surgeon. In the case in question, however, the Grand Duke recommended that two persons be sent: a doctor and a "gentleman." The reason for this was that the Florentine court did not want the mission merely to ascertain health

30. ASF, Sanità, Partiti, b. 13, c. 22v (29 July 1652). How anxiously the Florentine magistrates were waiting for the Genoese answer to their letter of July 20 is shown by the fact that at their meeting of July 27 they decided to postpone any answer to the Genoese declaration of the thirteenth till they had learned the reaction of the Genoese to their new approach; ASF, Mediceo, b. 2327 (27 July 1652).

31. ASF, Sanità, Partiti, b. 13, c. 22v (30 July 1652).

32. When in 1649 an epidemic of typhus afflicted Genoa, both Florence and Milan sent doctors of their own health services to make sure that it was not plague. The foreign doctors were welcomed in Genoa in a spirit of solicitous collaboration: see ASF, Sanità, Negozi, b. 184, cc. 97 ff. (24 May 1649); c. 100 (27 May 1649).

conditions in Genoa. The Florentines realized that the current situation had come about because of a persistent climate of reciprocal suspicion between the two states and because of a lack of precise information. They also recognized that if preventive. measures of public health were to have any chance of success, they would have to be agreed upon, coordinated, and enforced by neighboring states through common action. With these thoughts in mind the Grand Duke and his councilors had developed the idea of a convention (*capitolazione*), to be agreed upon by Florence, Genoa, and the Holy See. The convention would bind the three powers to adopt common public health practices and measures in the three main harbors of the Tyrrhenian Sea—Genoa, Leghorn, and Civitavecchia. To guarantee the observance and enforcement of the measures agreed upon, each state would allow the other two to station one representative of their respective health boards in its main harbor: thus, in Civitavecchia there would be one health officer from Florence and one from Genoa; in Leghorn, one from Rome and one from Genoa; and in Genoa, one from Rome and one from Florence.[33]

As far as I know, the scheme of the convention just described has passed totally unnoticed by both general historians and historians of medicine—and yet it represented a revolutionary and enlightened idea which, in the interest of "the common health," envisaged international controls and the voluntary relinquishment of discretionary powers by fully sovereign states in the matter of public health.

As indicated above, these ideas were presented by the court to the Health Magistracy in Florence on July 30. Of course the Magistracy obliged, adopted the suggestion, and issued the orders for the immediate execution of the plan.[34] In agreement with the court, the magistrates appointed Dr. Monti and Signor

33. ASF, Mediceo, b. 2327.
34. ASF, Sanità, Partiti, b. 13, c. 22v (30 July 1652).

Silvestri to carry out the mission. Dr. Monti was the physician of the Health Magistracy of Leghorn. Signor Silvestri was a troubleshooter who had already been employed in similar circumstances.[35] The composition of the team clearly indicated that to the operation were attached not only a technical but also a diplomatic significance. Indeed the whole affair now began to move along two parallel lines: at the technical level, the Health Magistracy was supposed to maintain contact with its counterpart in Genoa and, it was hoped, reach the desired agreement; at the diplomatic level, the court alerted its diplomatic representative in Rome and instructed him to inform the Holy See of the Tuscan initiative.

Signor Silvestri and Dr. Monti left Leghorn by boat on the morning of Friday, August 2, and they arrived in Genoa on the evening of Saturday, August 3. In accordance with the local health regulations, their boat anchored at the new pier, by the lighthouse, in the outer part of the harbor where incoming vessels were held before being cleared by the health authorities (see Fig. 5). A small barge carrying a health guard approached the Tuscan vessel, and Signor Silvestri consigned to the guard a letter of credentials addressed to the Health Magistracy of Genoa. The Genoese magistrates obligingly convened on the morning of Sunday, August 4, discussed the matter, and decided to admit the Tuscans.

Pomp and circumstance were an important element of life in those days, and the visit of the two Tuscan envoys was consequently a matter subject not only to practical considerations but also to the rigid formulae of etiquette. The Tuscan envoys were first led into a room adjacent to the one where the Health Magis-

35. ASF, Sanità, Negozi, b. 184, c. 499 (8 September 1649); cc. 516 ff. (10 September 1649). The text of the instructions to Signor Silvestri can be found in ASF, Mediceo, b. 2327 (30 July 1652).

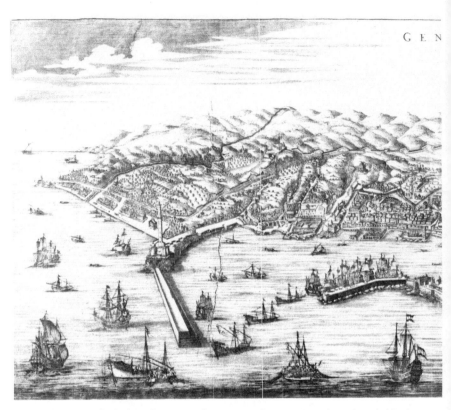

Figure 5. The harbor of Genoa in the seventeenth century. To the right, outside the walls and beyond the river, one can see the pesthouse. Map by Pierre Mortier

tracy convened and were left there while the syndic conveyed to the magistrates the purpose of the Tuscan mission. The magistrates then decided to admit Signor Silvestri to their presence. He was led into the main room, invited to take a seat, and asked to cover his head with his cap; he then explained in detail the purpose of his mission and the proposals of the Florentine Magistracy. The Genoese magistrates listened, grave and silent. After Signor Silvestri had finished his address, he was again shown into the adjacent room. When he was brought back to the magistrates' room, the magistrates were still there, as grave and silent

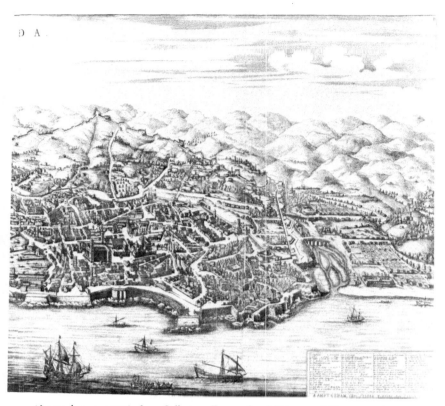

(Amsterdam, c. 1650), from Collezione Topografica del Comune di Genova, n. inv. 1182.

as before, and their chancellor spoke for them. He solemnly announced that, having discussed the matter, the magistrates had come to the conclusion that the Tuscan request to inspect the health conditions of the city was reasonable, and they authorized the two Florentines to visit the city and its harbor in the company of a physician, a surgeon, and the syndic of the Health Magistracy.

A rendezvous was arranged for the morning of Monday, August 5. The Genoese did not appear. They justified their absence on the grounds of urgent and unexpected business, although

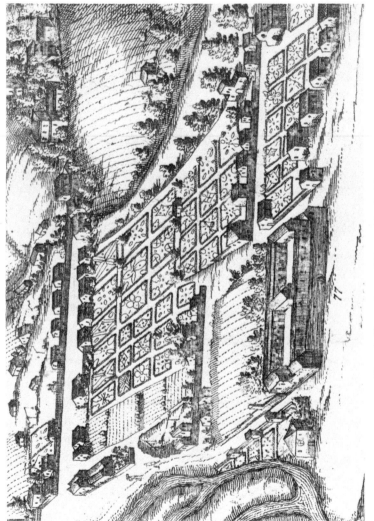

Figure 6. The pesthouse of Genoa. Detail of Figure 5.

Signor Silvestri suspected that they were instead making sure that everything was in order in the places that were going to be inspected. Whatever the reason for the delay, the three Genoese officials appeared after lunch and the inspection began. It lasted through Wednesday, August 7, and on Thursday, August 8, Dr. Monti was able to draft a report. It is a short but rather rare document which allows us to gain some insight into the health conditions of a large city of the time, when no epidemic prevailed.

Monday afternoon was spent in a visit to the pesthouse. The lazaretto was situated on the coast east of the town, quite outside the city walls (Fig. 6). The entrance to it was guarded by German mercenaries—a touch of efficiency which impressed the Tuscans. There were 293 patients in the pesthouse, divided into two separate groups. One group of 55 individuals was subject to *quarantena brutta* (ugly quarantine). The *quarantena brutta* derived its name from the fact that it was applied to people defined as *brutti* because they had caught the infection or had been in close and direct contact with infected people or merchandise. It meant complete isolation for 40 days or more, plus a further period of isolation described as "convalescence." This group included eleven sailors from the boat that had arrived from Sardinia and on which a sailor had died of plague, two other sailors who had attended the deceased one, eight passengers, one of whom had caught the plague but had recovered, and thirty-six among porters and disinfecters who had come in contact with the above sailors and passengers.

In another part of the pesthouse, in various rooms, the Tuscans found the other 238 inmates under the *purga di sospetto* (quarantine of suspicion). These individuals had not knowingly been in contact with infected people or merchandise, but they had either developed strange fevers or had come from areas where cases of plague had been reported. The Tuscan envoys noticed sixteen men in this group who had returned to Genoa

from Maremma and were suffering from "ordinary fevers."
Maremma was part of the Grand Duchy of Tuscany. It was a
vast region but sparsely populated because of the prevalence of
malaria, which was endemic in the plains of Tuscany. Seasonal
agricultural workers from neighboring states such as the Republic
of Genoa and the Duchy of Modena regularly went to Maremma
during the summer months, attracted by the relative shortage of
local labor—and they regularly caught the disease. In Tuscany
malaria was regarded as a common nuisance, and the two Tuscan
envoys were rather surprised to find that in Genoa people return-
ing from Maremma with such "ordinary fevers" were quarantined in the pesthouse; they took the fact as further evidence that
the Genoese Health Magistracy "abounded" in precautions.

Upon the arrival of the inspection party, all the inmates in the
pesthouse were ordered to take off their clothes. Dr. Monti
visited each of them individually—first those under *quarantena
brutta* and then those under *quarantena di sospetto*—and found
no pathognomonic signs of plague on anyone.

The following day, Tuesday, August 6, was devoted to visiting the two main hospitals of the city, the Spedale Maggiore
(Main Hospital) and the Spedale degli Incurabili (Hospital of the
Incurables). In both hospitals the men and women were kept in
separate quarters. In the Main Hospital the patients were classi-
fied into two main groups: those "with fevers," who were
treated by the physicians, and the "patients for the surgeon"—
namely, people suffering from wounds, skin ulcers, sores, and
abscesses. The distribution of patients in the Main Hospital was
as follows:

	Male	Female	Total
Patients treated for fevers	92	152	244
Patients for the surgeon	38	31	69
Children (with fevers)	0	45	45
Convalescents	14	44	58
	144	272	416

The term "fever" covered all kinds of symptomatic pathological conditions, and the wide use of it as a nosological and diagnostic term reflected the fundamental ignorance of the medical profession.

The number of patients at the Hospital of the Incurables was noticeably greater than at the Main Hospital: 698 compared to 416. Dr. Monti grouped the patients into seven main categories. Retaining those categories (as well as the diagnoses), one can summarize Dr. Monti's data as follows:

	Male	Female	Total
Patients suffering from paralysis, apoplexy, cancer, dropsy, and tuberculosis	152	256	408
Languids	26	32	58
Lunatics	39	33	72
Epileptics	19	42	61
Crippled	5	10	15
Syphilitics treated with diet	3	6	9
Syphilitics treated by purging	0	15	15
Children	30	30	60
	274	424	698

In both hospitals the females outnumbered the males in practically every category with the exception of the categories of lunatics and "patients for the surgeon" at the Main Hospital; the latter included individuals suffering from wounds inflicted by weapons or resulting from accidents at work. Taking both hospitals together, the females accounted for 62 percent of the total number of inpatients.

Genoa had a population of some 80,000 people in 1652. The 1114 patients in the two hospitals represented about 1.4 percent of the population. To assess the meaning of this figure, one has to keep in mind that (a) as repeatedly stated in the documents of the time, Genoa's population was then in a state of good health; (b) only the poor went to the hospitals,[36] and (c) not all patients admitted to the hospitals were necessarily inhabitants of the city; some actually came from the surrounding countryside.

But let us return to our two Tuscan envoys. By mid-afternoon on that Tuesday they had finished their visit to the hospitals, and they began the inspection of the harbor. Some 80 vessels were docked there, with 553 sailors.[37] Dr. Monti and Signor Silvestri spent the rest of Tuesday and the whole of Wednesday moving from one boat to the next; by Wednesday night the inspection was over. Dr. Monti's report gives a detailed list of all the boats and their crews, but considering the numbers involved, one can hardly believe that the visit was very thorough. One can legitimately suspect that the two envoys were happy and satisfied to be told by the ships' masters and/or the ships' surgeons that everything was in good order.

On Thursday morning, August 8, Signor Silvestri and Dr. Monti reported to the health Magistracy in Genoa. As one would expect, pomp and ceremony prevailed once again. The two envoys were admitted to the room where the magistrates were sitting. The doctor spoke first. He declared that he had visited the pesthouse, the hospitals, and the harbor and had found no evidence of contagion. Then Signor Silvestri spoke. He said that the inspection by Dr. Monti had dissipated all possible doubts about health conditions in the city and he added that the quarantines and other health regulations were being enforced so diligently that one could feel very confident about the future. Thus, he concluded, there should be an immediate and formal repeal of the suspensions, and each state should open its borders to the other.

36. By the end of the eighteenth century, out of some 5,000 people who died annually in Milan, less than 2,000 died in the hospitals, and of these more than 500 were abandoned children (Zanetti, "La morte a Milano").

37. The figures quoted are derived from the report of Dr. Monti. Signor Silvestri in his report speaks of 93 ships and 561 sailors.

The magistrates listened gravely, and after Signor Silvestri terminated his speech, the two envoys were invited to retire to the adjacent room. They were recalled a few minutes later. The magistrates were still there, and their Chancellor spoke for them. The magistrates, he said, were happy to hear that the Tuscans had found that health conditions in Genoa were good; the Magistracy had known this all along. If the Tuscans had come to Genoa at an earlier date, they would have reached the same conclusions, and all subsequent troubles would have been avoided. The magistrates were going to prepare a written answer for the Magistracy in Florence. Thereupon the two envoys were again invited to retire.

And retire they did. But Signor Silvestri was not at all pleased. Totally bewildered, he rushed off to Signor Giovanni Antonio Spinola, a Genoese nobleman who maintained good relations with Florence, and asked him to find out what had been meant by the magistrates' "very dry answer." Could the suspensions be considered lifted? The Florentine authorities had invisaged a formal and mutual declaration of a return to normalcy in the relations between the two powers. Could such a declaration be made? And when and in what terms? And what about the proposal of a convention among the Grand Duchy, the Republic, and the Holy See? On all these relevant questions, the magistrates had said absolutely nothing.

Signor Spinola contacted his friends in the Magistracy and then reported to Signor Silvestri that a letter addressed to Florence was in fact being drafted, but it did not contain one iota more than what had already been said orally. This was too much for Signor Silvestri, who went back to the syndic of the Magistracy, asking bluntly for a more specific answer. The syndic told Silvestri that he would deliver the letter in the afternoon. Signor Silvestri answered that he was not interested in the letter. Instead, would the syndic tell the President of the Magistracy that, having received "such a dry answer," he, Silvestri, was afraid that he had not made himself clear about the purpose of the mission, and that he therefore requested another audience.

The following morning, Friday, August 9, Signor Silvestri and Dr. Monti were again admitted into the presence of the Magistracy, and Signor Silvestri went directly to the heart of the matter: ''In the previous audience I said succinctly that it was possible mutually to restore trade and open the borders. On this point, your Lordships did not give me a specific answer, and consequently I had no opportunity to be more explicit. I can now add that I have authority from Florence to determine with you on what date to remove restrictions and put all [our agreements] into immediate effect.'' The magistrates listened gravely and silently and this time, as an act of exceptional courtesy, the President spoke for them instead of the Chancellor. He said: ''These Lordships have understood everything very well, and they will give an answer.'' That was all. Signor Silvestri and Dr. Monti were asked to leave the room; they were soon joined by the syndic, who informed them that they would receive a written answer in the afternoon.

The letter was delivered by the Chancellor, who informed Silvestri that it did not contain anything that Silvestri did not already know. In a friendly mood, however, he confided to Signor Silvestri that the magistrates thought that because the Florentines had been the first to suspend trade, they ought now to be the first to reopen it ''without negotiated declarations.'' He added that once the Florentines had repealed the suspensions, the Genoese would do the same. Silvestri was not convinced. He refused to accept the letter and pressed the Chancellor to go back to the President and ask him to put in writing the considerations expressed by the Chancellor. The latter obliged, but returned a little later with the same letter and advised Silvestri: ''Go; open the passes, and you shall see corresponding actions on our side.'' Silvestri had lost his reserve of patience and gruffly answered: ''I cannot force the will of the magistrates, but I tell you that in my opinion this is not the way to become reconciled.'' He took the letter and left the Chancellor. But he did not go back to his boat. Signor Silvestri was as suspicious as he was stubborn. He now suspected the Chancellor of duplicity, so he went back to Signor Spinola and pressed him to contact the magistrates once more and ask them for a specific answer. It was a futile effort, because the Chancellor had been sincere, and the Genoese magistrates were not the kind of people who would change their minds under the pressure of sheer persistence. Signor Spinola returned to Signor Silvestri empty-handed, and he too advised Silvestri not to lose any more time.[38]

The official report by Silvestri to the Grand Duke is dated August 14, but in all likelihood the Grand Duke by the thirteenth had already been briefed orally about the outcome of the mission. Officially he ignored the haughty posture of the Genoese, and even before his Health Magistrates met to discuss the matter, he wrote to his ambassador in Rome, instructing him to notify the Pope that it had been ascertained that health conditions in Genoa were good and that he planned to reopen trade with that city and her dominions. The Florentine Magistracy met on August 18, gladly concurred with the Grand Duke, and hastened to inform Genoa that orders were being issued to reopen the borders and renew trade.[39] The ordinance was published on August 19 in all cities of the Grand Duchy, and on the same day copies were dispatched to Milan, Venice, Ferrara, Mantua, Parma, Moderna, Ancona, and Bologna.[40] Genoa answered on August 23. It acknowledged the steps taken by Florence, though not without some further bickering about the way the Florentines had presented the facts in their ordinance of August 19. At any rate, on that same day, August 23, the Genoese issued an ordi-

38. For the account of this entire episode, see ASF, Mediceo, b. 2327.
39. ASF, Sanità, Partiti, b. 13, c. 23v (18 August 1652).
40. ASF, Sanità, Negozi, b. 187, cc. 562, 565; ASF, Sanità, Copialettere, b. 65, c. 22.

nance to reopen their harbors and territories to Tuscan travelers, merchants, and merchandise.[41]

Thus, by August 23 the situation was normalized between the two powers. The Florentines were now, however, determined to pursue their scheme of a convention among the Italian states along the Mediterranean Sea in order to standardize health regulations in their harbors.

On August 28 the Florentines wrote a letter to Genoa to acknowledge the Genoese repeal of the suspension of Tuscany, and they seized the opportunity to express their views—stating specifically that they "deemed it necessary that the various powers proceed in concert [di concerto] in the adoption and enforcement of measures regarding incoming vessels from areas either affected by the plague or suspected of it." According to the Tuscans, an agreement would have to cover such points as "how to receive such vessels, how to quarantine them, which merchandise to consider susceptible of infection and which not." They emphasized that a standardization of health measures would help to eliminate the frequent complaints of merchants and sea captains that health regulations were more strict and costly in one harbor than in another.[42]

It was a sensible letter, written in a frank and amiable tone, and it contained sensible ideas. Genoa answered on September 5: "We cannot but approve the wish to proceed united also in order to eliminate the occasion for the complaints we often hear that more leniency is practiced in Leghorn than here." Clearly the Genoese never missed an opportunity to be censorious. After that rather forbidding opening, however, their letter continued in a more agreeable tone. They assured their Florentine colleagues that they would not fail to concur with the Tuscan proposals;

41. ASF, Mediceo, b. 2327 (23 August 1652); ASF, Sanità, Negozi, b. 187, c. 593.
42. ASF, Mediceo, b. 2327 (28 August 1652).

they were pleased to inform Florence of the health regulations practiced in Genoa's harbor, and to this effect they enclosed a detailed memorandum; moreover, they declared that they were willing to consider all suggestions to complement their existing regulations "in order to fix up the whole and ensure the common health"—adding, however, that once a common set of rules was agreed upon, "there shall be no need mutually to keep monitors [in each other's harbors], since one party will have no doubts about the other party's observance of what has been agreed upon."[43]

The memorandum was couched in strictly pragmatic terms. There is no reference in it to general principles. Health regulations were described with specific reference to those areas which were effectively banished or suspended at the time the memorandum was compiled (see Appendix B). Thus the expression "proceed in concert" meant not only the adoption of a similar set of rules in the two harbors but also the stipulation that if and when one of the two parties would banish or suspend an area, the other party would automatically follow by virtue of the agreement.

On September 10, the Florentine Magistracy hastened to acknowledge receipt of the memorandum, and one week later, on September 17, having ascertained what the practices were in Leghorn, the Magistracy passed the information on to Genoa, noting not without satisfaction that the health authorities in the two harbors substantially followed the same practices, and that what differences existed were negligible and could easily be eliminated. The Florentine magistrates expressed their confidence that their Genoese colleagues would agree to the immediate application of the agreement, and concluded that "so long as we do not hear from you to the contrary we shall undertake to have assurances that the same or similar diligence is used in

43. ASF, Mediceo, b. 2327 (5 September 1652). See also Ciano, *La Sanità Marittima*, pp. 96 – 97.

Rome and Naples.'' Thus, as the letter indicates, the plan of the Florentines had in the meantime become more ambitious; it now included among the possible participants not only Florence, Genoa, and Rome, but also Naples.

Genoa answered promptly, three days later, on September 20. It gave full assurance of its intention to ''proceed in concert'' and expressed the wish to be informed promptly if Florence ''succeeded in inducing Rome and Naples to do the same.''[44]

Thus the *concerto* between Genoa and Florence had become a reality, but the task of inducing Rome and Naples ''to do the same'' was not going to be an easy one. One should keep in mind that while the Health Magistracies of Northern Italy had for a long time corresponded regularly among themselves, Rome and Naples had not been part of the ''corresponding'' circle.[45] The Florentine ambassadors in Rome and in Naples therefore had a double task: the *concerto* did not imply solely the adoption of the same set of rules established by Genoa and Florence; it also implied the commitment to regular and continuous correspondence by virtue of which each of all parties involved would share information and act together in the banishment or suspension of other states.

In the Holy City, Monsignor Scotti, Commissioner for Public Health, expounded to his colleagues the text of the convention agreed upon between Genoa and Florence, and had it approved. As to the establishment of a regular correspondence between Rome and Florence, the decision was that Monsignor Farnese, Archbishop of Patrasso and Governor of Rome, would be in charge of it and that he would limit himself to answering mes-

44. For greater detail on these communications, see Appendix B.
45. The point was made also by the Florentine Ambassador in Naples who, on August 20, 1652, wrote that the local Health Magistracy "non é solito carteggiare" [does not usually exchange correspondence] with the Health Magistracy in Florence (ASF, Mediceo, b. 2327).

sages from the magistrates in Florence, with the concession of addressing them with the title *Illustrissimi*.

In Naples the results were even more meager. In the opening move, the Florentine Ambassador approached the Regent on the point of correspondence. The Regent's answer was one of complete skepticism. He had no faith whatsoever in the local health board, which, as he explained, was composed of only two persons, a nobleman and a commoner who actually "bought" their position—the implication being that they paid themselves back through bribery. The Regent suggested that Florence should communicate directly with him, but please not to bother His Excellency with letters; the Ambassador could drop in when necessary and brief him orally.[46]

Having failed on this point, the Ambassador returned a few days later and presented the Regent with a copy of the convention agreed upon by Florence and Genoa. The Regent assured the Ambassador that Naples followed the same practices, but he also hinted that Naples, being a Spanish dominion, could not proceed in concert with Genoa and Florence when it was question of banishing or suspending Spanish territories, although he assured him that "diligent" precautions would be taken.

Thus the effort to bring Rome and Naples into the *concerto* was far from being successful. Genoa and Florence applied the *concerto* with determination and good faith, but there too the *concerto* lasted only a few years: in 1656–57 a disastrous epidemic of plague in Genoa forced Florence to banish her partner and put an end to the cozy relationship. Nevertheless, their short-lived *concerto* represented an early and quite remarkable chapter in the history of international health cooperation. Almost two centuries had to pass before something similar was tried again—when, prompted by the cholera scare, the first International Sanitary Conference opened in Paris on July 23, 1851.

46. ASF, Mediceo, b. 2327.

The conference gathered together delegates from not two but eleven countries. As for results, it yielded much less than the Genoese-Florentine negotiations of 1652. The delegates of the eleven nations took six months to achieve virtually nothing. From a practical standpoint, the Conference of 1851 was a fiasco. Its importance resided in the fact that, as one modern medical historian put it, ''The Conference established the principle that health protection was a proper subject for international consultation.''[47] As we have seen in the previous pages, that principle had been recognized centuries earlier by the Italian Renaissance states.

47. N. Howard-Jones, *Scientific Background*, p. 16.

CHAPTER 3

The Balance-Sheet of a Plague Epidemic: The Case of Pistoia in 1630–31

Coming from the north, the plague arrived in the Grand Duchy of Tuscany in the summer of 1630 and spread in the course of the autumn. The sequence of events is fairly clear: in the month of July a few persons died, allegedly of plague, in Trespiano, a small village a few kilometers north of Florence (see Fig. 7). According to the Health Deputies of the time, the plague had been brought to Trespiano by a man who, violating the sanitary cordon, had been on a business trip to the infected city of Bologna. In August suspicious deaths were recorded in the neighboring village of Tavola and in Florence itself.[1] On September 1, the plague made its appearance in Monte Lupo, 28 kilometers west of Florence, on the busy road to Pisa.[2] By September 19, the plague was recognized in Prato, about 20 kilometers northwest of Florence, on the road to Pistoia.[3] Before the end of the month the plague had reached Pisa.[4]

Unlike Florence and Leghorn, Pistoia did not have a permanent health board. Thus, about the middle of April 1630, when horrible news kept flowing in about the ravages caused by the plague in Northern Italy, the General Council of the city ap-

1. See ASF, Sanità, Rescritti, b. 37, cc. 20, 139, 144.
2. Cipolla, *Faith, Reason, and the Plague*, p. 16.
3. Cipolla, *Cristofano and the Plague*, p. 42.
4. Battistini, *Le epidemie in Volterra*, p. 45.

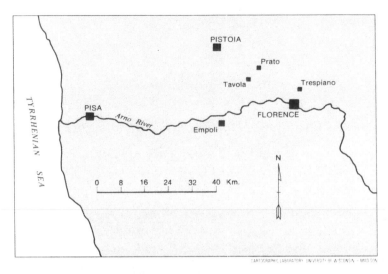

Figure 7. The Arno Valley.

pointed six gentlemen to the position of Health Deputies.[5] Understandably, the first measure taken by the newly appointed Deputies was the creation of a sanitary cordon around the city: guards were stationed at the gates and restrictions were placed on the movements of people and merchandise. Toward the end of April, the Health Deputies of Pistoia received an ordinance issued by the Central Health Magistracy in Florence, in which the Florentine authority recommended that, as a preventive measure, all cities of the Grand Duchy keep their streets as clean as possible. That was wise, and the Deputies of Pistoia acted accordingly.

The instructions and advice from the Florentine Magistracy were both numerous and continuous and covered much ground. But the Health Deputies of Pistoia did not want to risk overlooking any measure that could be of some use, and thus on

5. Salvi, *Delle historie di Pistoia*, p. 255. In this history of Pistoia, Father Salvi deals extensively with the measures taken by the local Health Deputies to fight off the plague, but the information he provides is largely inaccurate.

April 30 they consulted with four of the five local physicians. The advice they received throws light on the helplessness of medical science in the face of the plague in those days. All that the physicians could recommend was a prohibition on silkworms and on the production of raw silk within the city. Silkworms produced foul odors, and since the doctors thought miasmas were the cause of the plague, it is not surprising that they regarded silkworms with suspicion. (One only wishes that fleas and rats had also produced intolerable smells.) In Pistoia many people made a living by producing silk, and the measure recommended by the physicians would have severely affected the local economy; but the Deputies did not want to take chances, and they followed the physician's advice.

In the course of time the Health Deputies took other drastic measures. On July 19, on the advice of the local physicans, they resolved that no sick person would be admitted into the city unless he had previously been seen by one of the local doctors. On July 28, they expelled all foreigners, mountebanks, and Jews from the city, and on September 4 they renewed the ban on ''all those foreigners who are not subjects of the Grand Duke, with the exception of those who have home and family [in Pistoia].'' The idea was to relieve the crowded conditions within the city walls. At the end of July the Deputies refused to extend the annual livestock fair which was then taking place in Pistoia, and on August 16 they closed the city ''to all beggars and all poor people afflicted with any kind of disease.''[6]

The Deputies were not lacking in diligence. On August 23 they resolved ''that each one of them would go and visit the houses of Pistoia, especially the houses of the poor; and in the case they uncovered filth or anything whatsoever offensive to cleanliness, they would be empowered to have the filth removed

6. ASP, Provvisioni e Statuti, b. 554, cc. 17–22. When the epidemic broke out in October, the remaining beggars were assembled in one building and fed at the expense of the community; see Consoli Fiego, *Peste e carestie*, p. 95.

and to instruct the inhabitants to keep their homes as clean as possible. Moreover, if they were to find rotten wine, they could dispose of it.'' Their concern with cleanliness was most commendable; however, their preoccupation with rotten wine was at the same level as the physicians' preoccupation with silkworms. In the same vein, on September 4, the Deputies decided to discuss with the Bishop the possibility of having the fonts in the churches emptied of holy water for fear that it too could spread the contagion.

By the beginning of September, it was common knowledge that the plague had broken out in Florence and Monte Lupo. On September 9, the Deputies forbade all surgeons and barbers ''to go out of the city and bleed or treat anybody unless by special permission.'' The measure was obviously prompted by fear that knowingly or unknowingly the barbers and surgeons could possibly treat an infected person and bring the infection back to the city. The day after, September 10, all movements of people and merchandise to and from Florence were absolutely prohibited. However, weighty economic interests stood in the way of the public health requirements. Pistoia and its territory were one of the main suppliers of wine to Florence, and at the time of the grape harvest it was customary to bring the old wine to Florence in order to make room for the new wine in the cellars of Pistoia. The prohibition of September 10 had to be temporarily suspended only a few days after it had been decreed; the gates were temporarily reopened and people of all extraction swarmed back and forth between Pistoia and Florence.[7]

The Health Deputies grew increasingly nervous. They sensed that the circle was closing. On September 12 they wrote to the Grand Duke that ''so far Pistoia and the surrounding countryside have enjoyed perfect health,'' but considering the general

7. ASF, Sanità, Negozi, b. 150, c. 1386 (29 September 1630).

situation, they felt they had to take "stronger preventive measures, proportionate to the current perils." They estimated that public health expenditures would cost the city administration some 1000 scudi a month, and they therefore requested the authorization to borrow 9500 scudi in case of need. (We shall return to these figures later.)

On September 19, the plague was identified in nearby Prato. The circle continued to close, and the Health Deputies of Pistoia prepared for the worst. On the twenty-seventh they set up a pesthouse in a building two miles outside the city gates, on the road to Lucca,[8] and they appointed Dr. Stefano Arrighi, physician, and Master Francesco Magni, surgeon, to serve there. The two men were instructed to set up residence outside the walls of the city. The physician would receive a salary of 10 lire a day—that is, 43 scudi a month—while the surgeon would receive 15 scudi a month—that is, approximately one-third the physician's fee. Additional compensation was granted to both men for the use of a horse.

Then the circle closed. On the eighth of October the plague was reported in one house in Pistoia, and two days later another house was declared infected.

The Health Deputies were not medical men. They were administrators, and the proper and efficient use of the funds available was one of their main concerns. On the same day that the first case of plague was uncovered in Pistoia, they resoved to deposit all their present and future funds with the Rospigliosi Bank of Pistoia, and they agreed that all expenditures by the health board would have to be made not in cash but through the bank on the orders of at least two of the Deputies. Two days

8. The building had served as a hospital in previous centuries. It was known under various names—hospital of Santa Maria Maggiore or della Gronda or di San Lazzaro. It had ceased to serve as a hospital in the sixteenth century; see Consoli Fiego, *Peste e carestie*, p. 96.

later, in order to provide for the urgent expenditures which would not suffer any delay, and at the same time to maintain constant and prompt information on the financial situation, the Deputies appointed a *Provveditore* (general manager) in the person of Nofri Nencini.[9]

The Deputies' way of dealing with the Church bears the same imprint of practicality. As the epidemic progressed, the Deputies had to adopt more severe and stringent measures, thus antagonizing an increasing number of people. As Health Deputies, they had all the power they needed to overcome the resistance of ordinary citizens, but if clergymen violated the health ordinances, the Deputies could not proceed against them. The sensitive and delicate relationships between State and Church were at stake, and health officers in the Grand Duchy knew all too well that before proceeding against a clergyman, they had to present the case to the Grand Duke and obtain his personal license. In the rosiest of all hypotheses, that would mean long delays which would be intolerable when immediate action was necessary.

I have described elsewhere the ordeals that Health Deputies of the Grand Duchy suffered because of the opposition and antagonism of the clergy.[10] In a rather unorthodox procedure, the officers of Pistoia decided to take the bull by the horns. On October 8 they resolved to contact the local Bishop and obtain from him ''license to lock up and quarantine the houses of clergymen whenever a case of suspicious contagion occurred in them''; on November 4 they resolved to address the Bishop with another petition ''asking him to appoint four clergymen who would participate with the Health Deputies in their meetings, so that with their license and in ways agreeable to them it would be possible to proceed against priests and friars in

9. See ASP, Provvisioni e Statuti, b. 554, for the dates indicated.
10. Cipolla, *Faith, Reason, and the Plague.*

56

matters of public health without being obliged to have recourse every time to his Highness and most Serene Grand Duke.'"[11] The Bishop obligingly consented.[12]

Among the Health Deputies of the various cities and villages, those of Pistoia distinguished themselves for diligence and dedication. The Marquis Luigi Vettori, a General Commissioner, reported to Florence in the spring of 1631 that the Deputies acted nobly, "without regard to risks to ther persons, personal expenses, and other inconveniences.'"[13] All available evidence supports the judgment of Signor Vettori. In assessing results, however, one has to keep in mind that the Deputies operated with severe constraints. One constraint was the medical ignorance of the time, which meant that the Health Deputies as well as the medical men had to fight in the dark, waging an impossible battle against an invisible enemy. A second constraint was of an economic nature. Preindustrial societies were fundamentally poor, and resources available to the Health Deputies were severely limited. One should add that Tuscan administrators were traditionally parsimonious, and the Health Deputies of Pistoia were no exception.

As indicated above, the local Deputies were supervised by a General Commissioner, the Marquis Cavalier Luigi Vettori, who had been sent to Pistoia from Florence. Judging by his correspondence, Signor Vettori was an unusually diligent and meticulous man. Toward the end of the epidemic which struck the territory under his jurisdiction, he addressed a statistical report to the Health Magistracy in Florence which is admirable both for the information it contains and for the clear form in which it is presented. The Magistrates in Florence were im-

11. ASP, Provvisioni e Statuti, b. 554.
12. Salvi, *Delle historie di Pistoia*, p. 257.
13. ASF, Sanità, Negozi, b. 157, c. 564 (18 May 1631). See also cc. 596 ff. (19 May 1631).

Table 3.1. Number of Admissions and Deaths in the Pesthouses of Pistoia during the Epidemic of 1630–31

	Patients admitted to the pesthouses			Patients deceased in the pesthouses		
	From the city	From the country-side	Total	From the city	From the country-side	Total
1630						
October	2	29	31	1	5	6
November	15	126	141	7	65	72
December	35	151	186	21	79	100
1631						
January	11	68	79	6	35	41
February	13	31	44	11	14	25
March	10	57	67	4	26	30
April	21	49	70	12	28	40
May	4	107	111	4	47	51
June	9	173	182	8	93	101
July	9	188	197	4	85	89
August	—	90	90	—	52	52
Total	129	1,069	1,198	78	529	607

Source: Report of Marquis Vettori, ASF, Sanità, Negozi, b. 161, c. 461 (14 September 1631).

Note: By the end of August the epidemic was practically over in the city, but it was not totally extinguished in the countryside. Only in the second half of November was Signor Nencini, *Provveditore* of the Health Deputies, in a position to inform Florence that in the whole district of Pistoia there were "only" three villages with a few infected homes (ASP, Sanità, b. 550 bis [22 November 1631]).

pressed, and while thanking Signor Vettori for the report, they complimented him by recognizing that ''it was done as it should be—namely, with punctual precision.''[14]

The report, which Marquis Vettori forwarded to the Magistracy in Florence on September 14, 1631,[15] was divided into two parts: one part related to the demographic aspects of

14. ASF, Sanità, Copialettere, b. 59, c. 67v (25 September 1631).
15. ASF, Sanità, Negozi, b. 161, c. 461 (14 September 1631). At present, the report is not attached to the letter; it is in ASF, Sanità, Negozi, b. 161, cc. 941 ff.

the epidemic, the other to its financial aspects. The story unfolds as follows.

Judging by the admissions to the pesthouses (see Table 3.1)[16] the epidemic developed rapidly during the months of October, November, and December. It subsided with the beginning of the new year. On January 13, the Deputies noticed that "the contagion has abated" and, parsimonious as they were, eleven days later they proceeded to discharge a number of people employed in their service and to reduce the salaries of those retained.[17] On March 25 Signor Vettori reported to Florence that "in the city there is not one case of infection and in the surrounding countryside as well as in the pesthouses outside the city the number of patients and convalescents is less than it has ever been. However, it does not seem that the contagion is over and the fear remains that it will break out again when the warm weather supervenes."[18] He was prophetic. In April and more conspicuously in May the epidemic flared up again and stayed through the summer (see Fig. 8).[19] As indicated in Appendix A, on the basis of what we know about the etiology of the plague and the role of the fleas as vectors of the pathogen, it is not difficult to explain the two-wave course of the epidemic.

The pesthouses outside the gates accepted patients not only from the city but also from the countryside. If one distinguishes between the two groups, one notices that whereas in the city the first wave of the epidemic was by far more severe than the second, the opposite was true for the countryside (see Table 3.1). The average number of patients admitted monthly from

16. As we shall see below, the original pesthouse was expanded in the course of time, and later a second pesthouse was opened.
17. ASP, Provvisioni e Statuti, b. 554.
18. ASF, Sanità, Negozi, b. 156, c. 4 (25 March 1631).
19. In the city the epidemic practically ended with the end of the summer, whereas in the countryside it lingered throughout the fall; see note to Table 3.1.

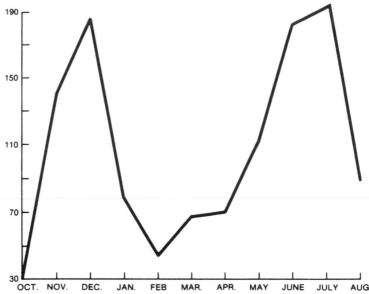

Figure 8. Number of patients admitted to the pesthouses of Pistoia from October 1630 to August 1631.

the city in the first five months of the epidemic (15.2 patients) was about double the corresponding average for the last five months (8.6 patients), while in the case of the countryside the average for the first five months (81 patients) was only two-thirds of the average for the last five months (121.4 patients). Clearly, in the first round the epidemic was centered on the city, whereas in the second round it ravaged the countryside.

As mentioned above, a lazaretto had been set up outside Pistoia on September 27. From the records of the health board we learn that a private house was first locked up in Pistoia on October 8, 1630.[20] In all likelihood, the first patients arrived in the lazaretto on that same day. What they found—or better yet, did not find—is reported in a letter which Dr. Arrighi hastened to dispatch in alarm that very same day to the Health Deputies:

20. ASP, Provvisioni e Statuti, b. 554, c. 27 (8 October 1630).

"Nothing we need is here; there are no bandages for bloodletting nor cloth for dressing tumors, and there are no attendants."[21]

That was just the beginning of the ordeals. By October 23, the Deputies were confronted with the fact that "the number of patients at the lazaretto keeps growing to such an extent that there is no room in it for all of them." Hard pressed, the Deputies hurriedly resolved to requisition "all houses situated in the same block as the lazaretto, as well as the houses facing it"; they also resolved to order twelve more beds for the hospital, and to make provisions that patients who recovered be promptly dismissed and sent to a convalescent home in order to make room for new patients in the lazaretto.[22] The resolutions were good, but the epidemic, though not particularly violent, kept running ahead of the Deputies. Whereas during the month of October, 31 patients were admitted to the pesthouse, in November the number rose to 141 (Table 3.1). On November 25, the Deputies resolved to look for another building to set up a second lazaretto.[23] They were still searching when they received a dramatic message from Dr. Arrighi on December 1:

Here the sick continually increase in number, and medication is lacking. We have sent repeated requests to the *Provveditore* and to the Hospital del Ceppo for cupping glasses, black soap, *conconi* for bloodletting, and other things, but nothing arrives, whence it follows that the disease undergoes little respite.

The general situation is very much affected by this, and the patients cannot be dismissed with the rapidity one would hope for.

Regarding linen and blankets: most of the beds are without sheets and have few blankets.

Regarding beds: the patients are five to a bed, to the detriment of the convalescent who, because of close contact with contagion, suffer relapses.[24]

21. ASP, Sanità, b. 550 (8 October 1630).
22. ASP, Provvisioni e Statuti, b. 554, c. 33 (23 October 1630).
23. ASP, Provvisioni e Statuti, b. 554, c. 44 (25 November 1630).
24. ASP, Sanità, b. 550 (1 December 1630).

The following day, December 2, the Deputies decided to turn to charity and ''go around in the city and collect blankets, mattresses, linen clothes, woolens, and other things to be used in the service of patients and attendants in the pesthouse.''[25] They also resolved that of the belongings seized in the homes of people who had died of plague, ''those which were not burned ought to be sent to the pesthouses.''[26] The measure was not an orthodox one, but scarcity left little room for orthodoxy. While the growing number of patients created one set of problems for the Deputies, the growing number of deaths created another. On December 2, in addition to the other resolutions, the Deputies decided to enlarge the cemetery next to the pesthouse, hire more gravediggers, and buy more lime.[27] They did not remain idle, but neither did the microbes. On December 12, Dr. Arrighi sent another dramatic message from the lazaretto:

> Twenty people, both men and women, are at the pesthouse waiting to go to the hospital at Capo di Strada [the convalescent home], but there are [new, clean] clothes for [only] six men and six women. I beg you to see to it that the rest of the clothes arrive so that they may all go to Capo di Strada.
>
> The number of patients in the pesthouse is increasing and there is no longer any place to put them, as they are lying four or five to a bed.
>
> We need vesicants and oils, and the Hospital del Ceppo says they have no more. And we also need straps to tie down patients who go out of their minds.
>
> In the Hospital at Capo di Strada there are twenty-one patients and only six beds . . . and they also complain of the food and bread which is so meager they say they cannot survive.[28]

The Deputies were caught between the devil and the deep blue sea. On the one hand, with the epidemic rampant, they were worried that not all infectious cases were being reported or

25. ASP, Provvisioni e Statuti, b. 554, c. 46 (2 December 1630).
26. ASP, Provvisioni e Statuti, b. 554, c. 50 (16 December 1630).
27. ASP, Provvisioni e Statuti, b. 554, c. 46 (2 December 1630).
28. ASP, Sanità, b. 550 (12 December 1630).

detected or that not all persons infected with the plague were being hospitalized. On the other hand, they were alert to the crowded conditions at the lazaretto and were worried that people suffering from ailments other than the plague would be admitted to the pesthouse. On November 4, 1630, they notified doctors, surgeons, and barbers that all medical men had "to report *in scriptis* [in writing] to the Chancellor [of the health board] all patients whom they treat daily and declare the nature of their ailments."[29] On the twenty-sixth of the same month, they resolved to hire a doctor and a surgeon to visit all those in the city afflicted with suspicious ailments. Obviously, the Deputies were most anxious to detect all cases of infection and dispatch the infected and their contacts to the pesthouses. However, on December 6, they decreed that no sick person could be admitted to the pesthouse unless he had been seen by the lazaretto physician, Dr. Arrighi, who had to ascertain that the patient was actually suffering from the plague.[30]

Dr. Stefano Arrighi was a young man of thirty years. He was the youngest among the five physicians living in Pistoia, a bachelor, and in normal times served as the community physician[31]—all, undoubtedly, reasons why he was chosen for the dangerous and unenviable assignment of serving in the pesthouse. Judging from his correspondence, the young doctor was a compassionate and very dedicated man. In June 1631 he was still alive, and he wrote a report to the Health Deputies on the regimen and treatments he used for the patients in the pesthouse:

> These poor wretches come to the pesthouse when the disease is far advanced, whence follows that they are extremely weak in regard to

---

29. The decision to notify the doctors was reached on October 30. See below, footnote 52.
30. See ASP, Provvisioni e Statuti, b. 554, for the dates indicated in the text.
31. Cipolla, *Public Health and the Medical Profession*, p. 119.

both their vital and animal forces. Consequently, I consider it good to refrain from bloodletting and giving purgative medicine, but recommend rather that immediately and then every other day they be given an ordinary enema.

Let them be fed with meals of good meat and eggs, withholding wine from them and giving them instead distilled spirit mixed with water.

I recommend rubbings and cupping glasses morning and evening, and when spots show on the skin they should be scarified for the first time.

I recommend that once a day the patients take eight drops of *olio contraveleni* [anti-venomous oil] with a little pimpernel water two hours before dinner.

In the morning at dawn everyone is to be given a glass of goat's rue water or vinegarish or pimpernel water, and it is also good to anoint the region around the heart, the stomach, and the pulses with *olio contraveleni* every six hours.

Application of hot concoction in the heart region should not be neglected either in the morning or in the evening, and during the day patients should often drink electuary of mulberry or conserve of citron.

It should also be arranged that fragrant herbs sprinkled with vinegar be kept throughout the hospital. And above all great care should be paid to cleanliness and purity.[32]

In his report the doctor showed a healthy dose of good, common sense. He took into serious consideration the poor physical condition of the patients at the time of their admittance to the hospital, and he chose to refrain from the common practice of phlebotomy. He recommended ''meals of good meat and eggs.'' ''Above all'' he recommended ''cleanliness.'' No one could argue with such recommendations. But the ministrations of the other standard drugs—including the highly reputed *olio contraveleni*, which was a disgusting concoction of boiled scorpions produced by the pharmacy of the Grand Duke—are witness to the fact that even at its best, medical treatment was

32. ASP, Sanità, b. 550 (1 June 1631).

worthless. The patients' chances of survival depended exclusively on the *vis medicatrix naturae*.

According to Signor Vettori, over the period October 1630 through August 1631, 1198 patients were admitted to the pesthouses, and of these 607 died (Table 3.1). The mortality rate was thus about 51 percent. I purposely use the expression mortality rate instead of fatality rate because owing to the unsatisfactory diagnostic facilities available at the time, it is far from certain that all patients admitted to the pesthouses were actually suffering from the plague. We saw above that the Health Deputies themselves had suspicions in this regard.

A mortality rate of 51 percent looks tragically high to modern eyes, but in fact it was not high at all. As the epidemics of plague of the nineteenth and twentieth centuries in India and Manchuria have abundantly demonstrated, among untreated patients suffering from bubonic plague leading to bacteremia, fatality rates range from 60 to 80 percent. The medical treatment practiced in the pesthouses at Pistoia, as we saw above, was of no practical value. The presence of some individuals suffering from other and less fatal ailments than the plague may have served to lower the average mortality rate, but if at the pesthouses the mortality was 51 percent instead of 60 or 80 percent, in my opinion the basic explanation has to be sought in another direction. The plague is a fast killer. In untreated patients death normally occurs within a period of three to six days from the onset of the illness. Patients who survive the seventh or eighth day have a good chance of recovery. It follows that if hospitalization is not prompt, a number of patients will die at home, and those who reach the hospital will represent a select and more resistant group. Differential mortality among the patients at the pesthouses in Pistoia supports this view. If one distinguishes between patients from the city and patients from the countryside, one finds that mortality among the former

65

reached the level of 60 percent, while among the latter it was only 50 percent. Hospitalization was obviously more prompt for those who lived in the city and who therefore died in greater proportion at the hospitals; of those who lived in more or less distant and isolated villages and hamlets, a greater proportion must have died before hospitalization. Signor Vettori himself states that the data of his report ''do not include some 500 persons who, in our estimation, must have died at their homes in those places of the district which are more distant from the city and the pesthouses.''[33]

If some of the patients who arrived at the pesthouses from the countryside had already passed the critical stage of the disease, they obviously had a greater chance of survival, and since the patients from the countryside represented almost 90 percent of the total number of admittances to the pesthouses, the relatively lower mortality of their group brought down the overall average mortality rate at the hospitals.

In the ordinary budget of a town like Pistoia, the only provisions for public health expenditures were for the salaries of the community doctors (one physician and one surgeon). When an epidemic broke out and extraordinary expenses had be be met, the Health Deputies had to look frantically around for funds. According to Signor Vettori, from October 1630 through August 1631 the Deputies were able to muster funds to the tune of ten thousand scudi.[34] Their main sources of financing were public revenues, charitable contributions, and loans. Public revenues, however, accounted only for the miserable sum of 250 scudi, which the Deputies were able to obtain from the board of highways and rivers and from the board of road pavement. By

33. ASF, Sanità, Negozi, b. 161, c. 461 (14 September 1631).
34. In Vettori's report the accounts are given in scudi, lire, and soldi; these related to each other as follows: 1 scudo = 7 lire, 1 lira = 20 soldi.

far the greatest part of their funds came from charity and loans, as shown by the following (rounded) figures:

	Scudi	Percent
Public revenues	250	3
Charity	4,585	45
Loans	5,275	52
Total	10,110	100

Whether measured as a percentage of GNP or by any other standard, charity plays a minimal role in industrial societies, and one modern economist felt justified in writing that ''charity and gifts are outside the logic of the system.'' Today welfare arrangements, pension funds, and state expenditures largely take care of social needs. Preindustrial European societies, however, operated in a totally different way, and charity was an essential part in the logic of their system. The figures quoted above provide a good illustration of this point.

Actually, by the seventeenth century, charity was highly institutionalized. Large numbers of public or semipublic institutions such as charitable trusts, religious societies among the laity, professional associations, hospitals, etc., were available to donors (mostly testators) willing to make bequests for charitable uses. Such institutions, originally endowed with more or less large estates by their founders, kept accruing their wealth through reinvestment of part of their income and through donations they received from all avenues of society. Administratively, they enjoyed a fair degree of autonomy, although they were often under some form of public control, and they had to dispense their resources for the charitable purposes indicated at their foundation and/or whenever the public need required it. The role and functioning of such institutions in Venice have been amply described by Brian Pullan in his massive work *Rich and Poor in Renaissance Venice*. In Pistoia, among the numerous institutions of this kind, the most important were the Opera di

San Jacopo, the Opera di San Giovanni, and la Sapienza.[35] According to Vettori, for the period October 1630 through August 1631 the three trusts put cash amounts of 804, 125, and 325 scudi respectively at the disposal of the Deputies. In addition, the Opera di San Jacopo provided 2150 *staia* of wheat, which at the going price were worth some 2320 scudi.[36] The charitable trusts were by far the largest donors. The other major donor was the Monte di Pietà, a public bank whose profits had institutionally to be devoted to charity. There were also the alms collected in the churches and some other miscellaneous sources. Altogether the total of charitable contributions was subdivided as follows (in round figures):

	Scudi
Charitable trusts	3,575
Monte di Pietà Bank	500
Alms collected in the churches	410
Miscellaneous	100
Total	4,585

Having looked at the health board's revenues, let us now look at its expenditures. By the end of August 1631, the Health Deputies had spent some 2200 scudi for wages and some 1200 scudi for miscellaneous items. They had spent about 405 scudi in rents for the buildings used as pesthouses and convalescent homes, 105 scudi to convert these buildings into hospitals, and 360 scudi to furnish them. The Health Deputies also had to provide nourishment for the patients in the hospitals, the beggars of the city, and the people quarantined in their homes, both in the city and in the countryside. For ''food'' the Deputies spent some 2300 scudi in cash,[37] and in addition, they gave away

35. On these institutions see Piattoli, *Guida storica e bibliografica*, Vol. 2, Part 1, pp. 44ff. and 127 ff.

36. On one occasion, the Deputies bought 328 *staia* of wheat on the market and paid 354 scudi, 4 lire, and 13 soldi. This calculates to 1.08 scudi per *staio*. One *staio* was equivalent to approximately 24.3 liters.

37. The 2300 scudi can be broken down into cash subsidies (1295 scudi),

2418 *staia* of wheat, which at the going market price were worth some 2600 scudi. Expenditures can thus be summarized as follows (in round figures): [38]

	Scudi	Percent
Food	4,900	53
Wages	2,200	24
Renting, fixing, and furnishing the hospitals	870	10
Miscellaneous	1,200	13
Total	9,170	100

The figures speak for themselves. As we shall see below, the Deputies employed a large number of people in their fight against the plague, and the list of items in the "miscellaneous" category is far from short. Yet the cost of providing food to the needy represented more than half of the total expenditures of the board. In part, this reflects a typical characteristic of a preindustrial society: wages were relatively low in relation to the price of food, and food was the major element in the composition of effective demand. In part, it reflects the particular conditions of the moment. The years 1628 and 1629 had been marked by widespread famine in Northern Italy; 1630 was not as bad a year as 1629, but it was still a year of mediocre crops. In 1630 the Health Deputies of Pistoia had to buy wheat, and they paid 7.5 lire (= 1.08 scudi) per *staio*. In "normal" years the price was about 4 lire. [39] Thus the cost of providing food to the needy was greatly inflated by the unusually high prices of grain.

Among the food expenditures one should include 6 scudi, 4 lire, and 13 soldi which the Deputies spent to buy goats. The

meat (441), wine (428), oil (87), salt (21), and miscellaneous (28). Of the cash subsidies, 843 scudi were given to the beggars, 379 to households quarantined in the city, and 73 to households quarantined in the countryside.

38. In addition to the expenditures mentioned in the text, the deputies loaned some 640 scudi to the small communities of the district for their expenditures on health-related matters.

39. Parenti, *Prime ricerche*, p. 7 of Appendix 1.

amount is so small in both absolute and relative terms that if it were a question only of its monetary significance, there would be no reason for mentioning it. There is, however, a pathetic quality attached to it that places it on a totally different dimension. Among the people dispatched to the pesthouses there were mothers still nursing their infants. Some of the mothers died, others were unable to feed their children because of the disease, and the Deputies were faced with the problem of nourishing the infants. Healthy wet nurses understandably refused to move to the pesthouses, and in those days there were no canned baby foods. So the resourceful Deputies bought goats to feed the infants with goat's milk. How many infants there were and how many survived we do not know.

We saw that wages amounted to some 2200 scudi. I should mention that the wage rates did not remain constant over the whole period during which the hospitals were in operation. The Tuscans were very careful administrators, and when the epidemic abated in January 1631—even though only temporarily—the Deputies immediately took advantage of the situation, dismissed some members of the staff, and reduced the wages of the others. The same procedure was adopted for those employed outside the pesthouses.[40] Furthermore, the physician served for only five months at the pesthouse whereas the surgeon and his assistant served for eleven; clearly the services of the physician were considered too expensive. At any rate, the outlay on wages was as follows:

	Scudi	Percent
Personnel in the pesthouses	1,280	58
Personnel outside the pesthouses	920	42
Total	2,200	100

40. For similar parsimonious procedures in nearby Prato, see Cipolla, *Cristofano and the Plague*, pp. 131 ff.

Of which:

	Scudi	Percent
Medical personnel	580	26
Paramedical personnel	279	13
Religious personnel	156	7
Administration	306	14
Health pass controllers	145	6
Gravediggers	260	12
Police force[41]	230	11
Miscellaneous	244	11
Total	2,200	100

It is impossible to determine the exact size of the task force under the command of the Health Deputies. Signor Vettori does not give precise numbers for certain categories such as trumpeters, messengers, guards, male nurses, laundrywomen, disinfecters, and the like. Moreover, many of these people might have been employed only temporarily. At any rate, Signor Vettori refers to 26 individuals and to 14 generic categories which subsumed two or more individuals each. It is not unreasonable to assume that at full strength the task force of the health board of Pistoia—the town had a population of some 8000—was made up of more than 55 to 60 people, in addition to the Health Deputies.[42]

The breakdown of total miscellaneous expenses is of interest because it shows us the broad front on which the Deputies operated.

After patients in the pesthouses had recovered from the infection, they were not sent back to their own homes but were instead dispatched to a convalescent home. Convalescent homes

41. This figure includes 40 scudi paid to the guards at the pesthouses.

42. In Prato, whose population amounted to some 6000 inhabitants, the task force under the command of the local Health Deputies amounted to about 25 men (see Cipolla, *Cristofano and the Plague*, p. 47).

were intended not so much to help the convalescents in their recovery as to keep them isolated for a further period after they had been removed from the ranks of the sick. It was generally believed that a convalescent could still be infectious for some time. This was a sound and correct idea, although in the absence of microscopy it was an ingenious intuition rather than a scientifically tested fact. The basic rule was that the longer the period of isolation, the greater the margin of safety.

In Pistoia the Deputies set up two hospitals for the convalescent: one for men and one for women. When convalescents were sent to these hospitals, the clothing they had worn during their illness was burned and new clothing was provided. This was wise even judging by our modern scientific standards, since the old clothing could harbor infected fleas or be impregnated with infectious fluids. But it was costly. When instructing the *Provveditore* that the patients dismissed from the pesthouses had to be provided with new clothing, the parsimonious Deputies never failed to recommend that this be done "at the least expense possible."[43] Moreover, the Deputies collected "shirts and clothing" from charitable contributions. Despite these efforts, providing the convalescents with clean clothing cost some 489 scudi.

The remaining items in the miscellaneous list are of minor economic significance, but three deserve to be mentioned because they throw light on some of the epidemiological ideas of that time.

People thought that epidemics originated from noxious miasmas and that rotting corpses corrupted the air. Consequently, the Health Deputies went out of their way to make sure that plague victims would be buried at a given depth under ground. At one point, the Deputies actually spent ten scudi "to

43. ASP, Provvisioni e Statuti, b. 554, c. 37 (4 November 1630), and c. 52 (25 December 1630).

raise the level of the earth above those buried in the cemeteries of the pesthouses.''

Although nobody thought in terms of fleas and microbes, it was believed that the personal belongings of infected people could spread infection. On December 16, 1630, the Deputies ordered that "the goods, utensils, and other things belonging to persons who died of contagion ought to be burned, and those which are not burned ought to be sent to the pesthouse.''[44]

Given the general level of poverty and ignorance, the majority of the people were not ready to share such concerns. Reporting on the people in the countryside, Signor Vettori wrote that "not only do these *contadini* [peasants] not take any precautions, but they also refuse to believe that the infection remains attached to the belongings of the infected.''[45] Poverty was so great in those days that people actually waited for someone to die to get hold of his personal belongings.

The Deputies at Pistoia reimbursed a number of "*artisti* [craftsmen and laborers] of the city for belongings of theirs which were burned" to the tune of 43 scudi; they also reimbursed some *contadini* to the amount of 59 scudi for the same reason. Both figures are quite modest, which indicates several possibilities: either the Deputies encountered resistance in their efforts to destroy infected objects; and/or the objects destroyed were of little value; and/or reimbursement did not cover the full value of the objects that were burned.[46]

Furs as well as carpets and woolens were dangerous because they could easily harbor infected fleas. As shown in Chapter 1, people recognized that these materials could be a source of contagion, but since they were totally ignorant of the etiology of

44. ASP, Provvisioni e Statuti, b. 554, c. 50 (16 December 1630).
45. ASF, Sanità, Negozi, b. 157, c. 126 (5 May 1631).
46. In nearby Prato the rule was to reimburse the owners 50 percent of the "just" value of the goods which were requisitioned and burned (see Cipolla, *Cristofano and the Plague*, p. 91, n. 1).

the disease, they misused a perceptive and intelligent observation to construct an inaccurate theory—namely, that furs, carpets, and woolens were dangerous because the pestiferous miasmas would stick to them more easily than, let us say, to marble, glass, or iron. From this erroneous induction, they drew another induction—namely, that dogs and cats because of their fur, and chickens and pigeons because of their feathers, could spread the contagion.[47] In line with what was done in other cities,[48] the Deputies of Pistoia spent more than three scudi to

47. Although they were adducing the wrong reasons, the people of the late Middle Ages and the Renaissance were not totally wrong to consider cats and dogs as possible sources of infection during an epidemic of plague. Some contemporary cases may illustrate this point.

In 1977, a 23-year-old Arizona mother became ill after her pet cat began to move in an uncoordinated way and to cough up blood. All three members of her family had handled the animal, but only the patient and her husband had looked in its mouth. The cat wandered away, was found dead a few days later, and *Yersinia pestis* was isolated from its tissues. At Atlanta, officials at the federal Center for Disease Control said the mother's pharyngeal infection with cervical lymph node involvement had resulted from droplet transmission for the cat.

Another case in which all evidence suggests transmission of *Yersinia pestis* from a domestic cat to a human occurred in September 1977 in Valencia, New Mexico.

In California, on September 7, 1977, a 48-year-old Bakersfield woman was admitted to a local hospital in a toxic and confused state with a one-day history of high fever reaching 106° F., headache, generalized aching, chills, weakness, nausea, vomiting, and diarrhea. Between September 2 and 5 she had stayed at a private campground four miles south of Tehachapi, California (elevation: 4000 feet), where she and her husband had slept in a trailer. No rodent die-off was evident to them or on subsequent investigation, but possibly she was exposed to fleas carried by a dog with which she had played; the dog belonged to another member of the group, had no flea collar, and was allowed to roam freely in the camp area. The patient sustained many insect bites on her lower extremities. A very tender left inguinal node measuring 4 × 5 cm was palpated. There were insect bites on the medial aspect of her left knee and right thigh. A smear of lymph node aspiration on September 8, 1977, with Wayson's stain yielded bipolar forms typical of *Yersinia pestis,* which was confirmed from cultures of the lymph node and blood at the Microbial Diseases Laboratory.

See U.S. Department of Health, Education and Welfare, *Morbidity and Mortality Weekly Report 26,* no. 41 (October 14, 1977): 337.

48. For Florence, see ASF, Sanità, Rescritti, b. 37, cc. 596 and 641; for Padua, Ferrari, *L'Ufficio della Sanità,* p. 119, n. 5; for Verona, Pellegrini, *Per la storia della lotta contro le epidemie,* p. 29.

have the dogs of the city caught and killed—and by doing so they unwittingly made life easier for the rats.

We saw above that the Deputies' total outlay over the period October 1630 to August 1631 amounted to 9170 scudi. Although the epidemic was over in the city by the end of August 1631, it was still lingering in the countryside. Thus the Deputies had additional outlays during the last months of 1631, but these additional expenditures could not have come close to the amount spent during the previous eleven months. The annual public revenues of the city of Pistoia at that time amounted to approximately 28,000 scudi. I do not believe we would be much off the mark if we assume that the total outstanding expenditures of the health board of Pistoia during the entire epidemic amounted to approximately 40 percent of the average annual public revenues of the city. Of course, this figure does not represent the total economic cost of the epidemic. To what was actually spent one should add what was not gained because of the interruption of trade and communication, but on this point we have no information.

The data that we have analyzed so far—both demographic and financial—relate to the whole operation of the health board, whose jurisdiction covered not only the city of Pistoia but also extended to the district. Unfortunately, we have no idea of the size of the reference population; moreover, the population in question was far from homogeneous, since it included both urban dwellers and peasants living in the plains, hills, and mountainous areas. In Signor Vettori's report there are, however, further demographic data which refer specifically to the population of the city, whose size we know from other sources. Let us then return to demography.

We have already briefly discussed the data regarding the admissions to the pesthouses during the period October 1630 to

August 1631. If we focus our attention solely on urban dwellers admitted to the hospitals, further considerations are possible.

In most Northern Italian cities in times of epidemic, a number of obstacles prevented the Health Deputies from confining all infected people and their contacts to the pesthouses—as most of them would have liked to do. First of all, they quickly ran short of space in the pesthouses, and we saw above that Pistoia was no exception. Another set of problems was raised by the fact that a pesthouse was—to say the least—a preview of hell, and people resisted being confined in it or having relatives confined in it. If the Health Deputies managed to break down the resistance of the poor, they encountered insurmountable difficulties when it came to people of consequence. One should also remember that the people of the Middle Ages and Renaissance had a totally different concept of hospitals from ours: a hospital was a place which offered hospitality to the needy poor, whether sick or not; it was not a place for those who were not in need of charity. Last but not least, once people had been quarantined in a pesthouse, they had to be provided for. It was true that poor people locked in their homes still had to be provided with food, but if people of means were quarantined in their homes, they were supposed to take care of their own needs. Normally a compromise was reached whereby as many as possible of the infected of the lowest orders and their contacts were confined to the pesthouses while the well-to-do were quarantined in their homes. Rationalizing on this common practice, the Deputies argued that the poor lived in crowded quarters, and thus it was imperative in their case to remove the infected. The well-to-do, it was argued, had abundance of space and rooms, and even if locked up together in the same house, the infected and the healthy could keep at a safe distance from one another.

In the case of Pistoia, we can clearly see how differential treatment broadly coincided with social and economic stratification because Signor Vettori took care in his statistics to distinguish between *cittadini* and *artisti*, the former being the well-to-do and the latter being the craftsmen and laborers. Considering only the patients from the city, we learn from Vettori's report that during the period October 1630–August 1631, there were 129 admissions to the pesthouse (66 males and 63 females), and all of them came from the class of *artisti*. No *cittadino* was confined to the pesthouse. Conversely, it is impossible to say whether all infected individuals from the laboring class were actually confined to the pesthouse.

In those days a person walking through a city struck by the plague would have noticed—among a number of unpleasant things—that many houses had their doors nailed shut or bolted on the outside and marked with a cross to warn passersby. During the day the residents would frequently appear at the windows to chat with the people in the street, implore the benediction of a passing priest, ask medical advice from a doctor, and—more often—lower baskets to the street below to have them filled with necessities. Occasionally, the body of a deceased person, instead of a basket, was lowered to the street. A house was locked by the health authorities whenever a death occurred that was linked to plague or when a case of plague infection was detected or reported. In the latter instance, the house was locked whether the patient was left in the house or sent to the pesthouse.

According to Signor Vettori, during the period October 1630–August 1631, the following numbers of houses were locked up in Pistoia:

Houses of the well-to-do	11
Houses of laborers to whom food was not provided	15
Houses of laborers to whom food was provided	99[49]
Total	125

49. For the 99 households of workmen who were poor and had to be provided with food by the health authorities, Signor Vettori reports that they contained 370 "mouths." This gives an average of 3.7 persons per house, but it should be considered that in most cases when a house was closed, one or more of the inhabitants either had died or had been sent to the pesthouses.

Table 3.2. Confinements and Deaths among the Population within the Walls
of Pistoia during the Epidemic of 1630–31

| | Patients from within the walls | | | | |
	Confined to the pesthouses	Deceased in the pesthouses	Deceased in the city	Total deceased from the city	Number of houses locked up in the city
1630					
October	2	1	—	1	13
November	15	7	7	14	19
December	35	21	10	31	25
1631					
January	11	6	3	9	6
February	13	11	4	15	14
March	10	4	4	8	5
April	21	12	1	13	8
May	4	4	2	6	7
June	9	8	5	13	13
July	9	4	3	7	13
August	—	—	2	2	2
Total	129	78	41	119	125

Source: See Table 3.1.

The monthly data on the number of houses locked up in the city
(Table 3.2, last column) confirm what we have already argued
on the basis of the monthly admissions to the pesthouses—
namely, that the epidemic occurred in two waves, and that in the
city the first wave (autumn and winter of 1630) was by far more
severe than the second (spring and summer of 1631). As Figure
9 clearly shows, the curve of the number of houses which were
locked up closely parallels both the curve of admissions to the
hospitals and the curve of deaths. The curve of deaths brings us
to the final problem—namely, the mortality due to plague
among the population of the city.

The data provided by Signor Vettori for the period October
1630–August 1631 can be summarized as follows:

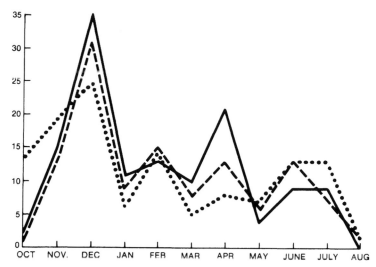

Figure 9. Comparison of number of houses locked up, admissions to the pesthouses, and deaths in Pistoia from October 1630 to August 1631. The dotted line shows the number of houses locked up, the solid line shows the number of patients from the city admitted to the pesthouses, and the dashed line shows the number of patients from the city who died, either at the pesthouses or at home.

	Deaths among well-to-do	Deaths among laborers	Total	Percent
In the pesthouses	—	78	78	66
At home	6	35	41	34
Total	6	113	119	100

The first thing to be observed is the proportion of people who died in the pesthouses, 66 percent. During the epidemic of 1610–11 in Basel (Switzerland) only 5 percent of the deaths occurred in the hospital. During the epidemic of 1630–31 in Carmagnola (Piedmont) and Prato (Tuscany), the corresponding figures were 24 and 27 percent respectively.[50] The proportion of

50. For Basel, see Platter, *Observationum,* pp. 321–22; for Carmagnola, see Abrate, *Popolazione e peste,* p. 86; for Prato, see Cipolla, *Cristofano and the Plague,* p. 147.

people who died at the hospitals was often very low because people resisted being confined to the pesthouses, cases of infection were not detected promptly, and when hospitalization was decided upon, it was often unduly delayed. The fact that the proportion was as high as 66 percent in Pistoia shows that the local Health Deputies went about their jobs with determination and efficiency. In view of what we know about them, this is not surprising; surprise is, however, in store from another quarter.

When we add those who died at the pesthouses to those who died at home, we reach a total of 119 deaths. As I have mentioned, at the outbreak of the epidemic the population of Pistoia must have amounted to some 8000 people. This leaves us with a mortality rate in the neighborhood of 1.5 percent—a figure which looks improbably low. Table A.3 (Appendix A) shows data relating to a number of other Italian towns during the epidemics of 1630–31 and 1656–57; we see that mortality rates ranged from 10 percent to 61 percent, with the greatest frequency in the 25 to 50 percent range. The mortality rate of 1.5 percent for Pistoia stands out as a unique and abnormal case.

Can we trust the information given by Signor Vettori? This is of course the first question that comes to mind. As we saw above, Signor Vettori gives two sets of monthly figures, one for the number of people who died in the pesthouses and one for the number who died in their homes. The latter total is also reported by other sources.[51] This suggests that Signor Vettori did not willfully belittle the phenomenon: clearly he reported information

51. The total of 40 deaths due to plague within the city of Pistoia was reported in the *Registro del Convento di Giaccherino* compiled in 1646. The register was consulted by A. Chiappelli, who passed on the information to Corradi (*Annali*, Part 2, Vol. 7, Appendix, p. 731, n. 7). The register was preserved at the Archivio di Stato di Pistoia but at present cannot be traced there.

Battistini, *Le epidemie in Volterra*, p. 44, erroneously maintains that in Pistoia there were 607 cases of death due to the plague. He misread Vettori's report. In the report, the figure 607 refers to the fatal cases in the pesthouses and includes the deceased patients from the countryside. Consoli Fiego, *Peste e carestie*, p. 104, quotes Battistini and makes the same mistake.

which was passed on to him. Thus the real question is whether there was underreporting of deaths from the plague.

There was no reason for the administrators in the pesthouses to underreport deaths. If underreporting occurred, it was in the city. When a death was recognized as due to the plague, the family of the deceased would have to be quarantined and all household items would have to be burned. Thus, pressures were no doubt put on doctors to report a fatal event as caused by an ailment other than the plague. The Deputies were alert to this possibility and were persistently on the lookout. As we saw above, on October 30 they resolved to notify all physicians, surgeons, and barbers in Pistoia that "they had to report *in scriptis* [in writing] to the Chancellor [of the health board] all patients whom they treat daily, and declare the nature of their ailments."[52] Fines for disobedience were established at 50 scudi for the physicans and 25 scudi for the surgeons and barbers. The ordinance was announced to the medical men individually, at their homes, on November 4. It is worth noting that the physicians, surgeons, and barbers were requested to report not only cases of plague, but all cases of sickness; obviously the Deputies were double-checking. But were their orders observed?

Signor Vettori clearly states that his figures concerning those who died in the city refer to "corpses which were sent out of the city to be buried at the pesthouse cemetery owning to a suspicion of contagion." To understand this notation, one has to keep in mind that the deceased were normally buried in the cemeteries of the churches within the walls of the city. However, in deference to the prevailing medical ideas about miasmas, the corpses of those who had supposedly died of plague were buried outside the walls for fear that if buried within the city, they would add to "the corruption of the air." Signor Vettori was perfectly right to count only those whose corpses had been taken to the com-

52. ASP, Provvisioni e Statuti, b. 554, 30 October 1630.

mon graves outside the walls as victims of the plague. If people died of plague within the city but the cause of death was not faithfully reported, their corpses were not dispatched to the common graves; such deaths would therefore not appear in Signor Vettori's figures; they would, however, appear by necessity in the parish books of the deceased, although obviously not as cases of plague. In those days Pistoia had 28 parishes. For 16 of them the books of the deceased for the years 1630 and 1631 have been preserved.[53] The sample is abundantly large and unbiased. I analyzed the books in question and found that the number of people buried in the cemeteries of the 16 parishes over the period March 1630–August 1631 was as follows:

Months preceding the epidemics:

March 1630	22 people buried
April	10
May	11
June	19
July	19
August	11
September	19

Months during which the epidemics prevailed:

October	15
November	13
December	15
January 1631	17
February	6
March	9
April	6
May	8
June	8
July	5
August	11

53. The registers are preserved in the Archivio della Curia Vescovile in Pistoia. The parishes are: Santa Andrea, Cattedrale, San Domenico, San Giovanni Evangelista Fuoricivitas, San Filippo e Prospero, San Ilario, San Leonardo, San Jacopino in Castellare, Santa Maria in Borgo Strada, Santa Maria Maddalena al Prato, Santa Maria dell'Umiltà, Santa Maria Maggiore, San Matteo, San Michele in Bonaccio, San Paolo, and San Salvatore.

Clearly, in relation to the level of mortality up to September 1630, the figures for the months during which the epidemic prevailed absolutely do not show any abnormal increase attributable to unreported cases of plague; on the contrary, the figures show a diminution of mortality obviously related to the fact that as people died at the pesthouses, there were fewer people left to die at home. Thus the medical men of Pistoia are cleared of the suspicion of underreporting. This brings us back to the figures of Signor Vettori, which can be put to another and decisive test.

The Tuscan census of 1622 listed 8386 people living within the walls of Pistoia. We do not know whether the population of the city grew between 1622 and 1628 or not, but we know that in 1629 the city had a heavy mortality because of the combined effects of an epidemic of typhus and a widespread famine.[54] At the beginning of 1630 the population within the walls must have been at or below 8000 people. As mentioned earlier in this chapter, just before the epidemic broke out, the Deputies expelled foreigners, mountebanks, and Jews from Pistoia. It is also possible that some people fled from the city.

In 1632, when the epidemic was over, another census was taken, and it was found that there were still 7721 inhabitants within the city.[55] These data suggest that the population losses in Pistoia due to the plague must have been *below* the 3.5 percent level.[56]

54. On the epidemic of typhus, see below, footnote 58. In addition to the parish books of the deceased, registers were kept in Pistoia in which the deceased were recorded in alphabetical order (ASP, Atti civili, Registri dei morti). Although these registers are not complete, it is significant that for 1629 they record a noticeably higher number of deaths than in the previous or in subsequent years: 359 in 1626, 422 in 1627, 472 in 1628, 787 in 1629, and 457 in 1630.

55. On the census data for Pistoia, see Del Panta, *Una traccia di storia demografica*, p. 45.

56. The losses would have amounted to 3.5 percent if the population at the beginning of 1630 had been 8000 (which is unlikely because of the mortality of 1629), if no people had been expelled from the city just before the outbreak of the plague (but we know that the ordinance for their expulsion was pro-

No matter how skeptical one tries to be, one has to admit that, at least as orders of magnitude, the data of Signor Vettori stand up to all possible tests. That solves one problem but opens up a more complex one: why did the plague cause such exceptionally minimal losses among the population of Pistoia in 1630–31? The Health Deputies acted with determination and diligence but, as I have already stated, they operated under the severe constraints of limited economic resources and incorrect medical theories. They did no more than most of their colleagues in communities which suffered losses on the orders of magnitude of 25–50 percent or more. The plague broke out in Pistoia in the late autumn; when the epidemic was gaining momentum, the cold weather of the winter months broke its vicious spiral; a second wave in the following spring never gained as much momentum. The seasonal timing of the events may thus have contributed to limit the damage. But the timing of the epidemic in nearby Prato was not different from that in Pistoia, and yet Prato suffered losses on the order of 25 percent.[57]

In the years 1628 and 1629 Pistoia had suffered from a combination of famine and epidemic. Could there have been a connection between the outbreak of an epidemic in 1628 and the exceptional mildness of the epidemic of plague two years later? If the epidemic of 1628–29 had been plague, the answer would undoubtedly be positive. But according to the doctors of the time, the epidemic of 1628–29 was typhus.[58] Broadly speaking, physicians were able to differentiate between typhus and plague. Admittedly, in the absence of microbiological observation, diag-

mulgated), if no people had fled from the city after the outbreak of the epidemic (which is unlikely), and if the number of newly born during the epidemic had equaled the number of those who died for reasons other than the plague (which is also unlikely).

57. Cipolla, *Cristofano and the Plague*, pp. 96–104.

58. On the epidemic, see Corradi, *Annali*, Vol. 3, p. 58, n. 1. With the outbreak of the epidemic, a physician of Pistoia edited a collection of writings on petecchial fever. The book, published in Pistoia in 1628 under the title *De febre maligna polydaedalae Medicorum epistulae*, is extremely rare today.

nosis could easily have been mistaken, but mortality in 1628–29 was relatively atypical for an epidemic of plague. If the killer in 1628–29 had been *Rickettsia prowaceki*, however, it is not clear how this could be related to the limited activity of *Yersinia pestis* in 1630. Lice may have died in great numbers during the typhus epidemic, but the main vector for the plague bacillus is the rat's flea. Our story ends with an epidemiological puzzle.

Appendixes
Bibliography
Index

The Plague in the Sixteenth and Seventeenth Centuries

Symptoms and Signs

Descriptions of the clinical symptoms of the plague are abundant for the centuries that followed the great pandemic of 1348. For the period and area covered by this book one finds accurate descriptions not only in the medical treatises by more or less famous scholars but also in the occasional writings and reports by obscure practitioners.

An anonymous physician from Bologna who sent a report on the epidemic of 1630 in that city to the Health Magistracy in Florence recorded that

> In some people very painful buboes appeared in the groin, and they showed in their center a tuberculum like a vetch seed. Some of the patients experienced anxiety, headache, thirst, small red spots which looked like flea bites on the skin, vomiting, and cloudy urine. . . . Besides those mentioned, the usual symptoms were delirium, dry tongue, and carbuncles in various parts of the body other than in the gland areas. Not all symptoms appeared in conjunction in all cases, but patients shared them in various degrees.[1]

Summarizing the observations of the members of the College of Physicians of Florence during the early phases of the epidemic of 1630, Dr. Antonio Pellicini recorded these symptoms:

> severe headache, anxious insomnia, mental derangement, burning thirst, lack of appetite, panting respiration, continuous anxiety, bitter

1. ASF, Miscellanea Medicea, b. 389.

vomiting, foul diarrhea, cloudy urine, very infelicitous pulse, burning face and eyes, dry and black tongue, unusual facial expression, unspeakable prostration. In addition, sometimes petechiae-like spots appear on the skin and also horrible pustules which contain water and are hideously black like carbuncles.[2]

During the epidemic of 1656–57 in Rome, a medical report recorded the symptoms as follows:

Onset is marked with very high temperature, very severe headache, bilious vomiting, sleepiness, occasional diarrhea, and cloudy, dark urine. If the above-mentioned signs did not appear on the first day, they did not fail to appear on the 2nd. Quite often on the 2nd day delirium also supervened. In many patients buboes and carbuncles appeared with the first attack of temperature. . . . In other patients buboes and carbuncles appeared on the 2nd, 3rd or 4th day. . . . Other and more numerous patients suffered from such a mild temperature that, according to Dr. Tomassini and Dr. Michele, they did not seem to run any temperature at all, but they experienced such severe prostration and such a loss of all natural vital and animal faculties that none reached the 3rd day, and yet they showed no exterior signs or petechiae on their bodies.[3]

For the sake of comparison I quote a description of the symptoms and signs of plague from a medical manual of our own times:

Onset, which often is abrupt, is marked by a slight chill, or repeated attacks of chilliness. Temperature then rises rapidly, usually to 103° F., but in severe cases may reach 106° F. The faces show fear and anxiety. Vomiting, thirst, unsteady gait, generalized pains, mental dullness and headache are the most frequent symptoms. The skin becomes hot and dry; pulse and respiration rate increase. The face becomes edematous and the conjunctive injected. Hearing may be impaired. Convulsion, stupor, or coma sometimes develop. Splenomegaly often is present. Involvement of the kidneys causes oliguria and albuminuria. Leukocytosis may be pronounced . . . Petechiae . . . can appear about the 3rd day. Gastrointestinal and pulmonary hemor-

2. Pellicini, *Discorso*, pp. 6–7.
3. Savio, "Ricerche, sulla peste," pp. 121–22.

rhage occur. Buboes (enlarged, painful, tender lymph nodes) usually appear between the 2nd and 5th days, and may suppurate.[4]

Diagnosis

Describing symptoms is one thing; diagnosing a pathological condition is quite another. The identification of plague and the admission of its presence were always subjects of much heated controversy. One has an embarrassment of choices in selecting instances of this recurrent fact. Dr. Ingrassia recorded that

> In 1535, while I was a student in Padua, a pestilence broke out in Venice and the doctors were unable to identify it. . . . In Venice again, in 1555, there prevailed a great diversity of opinions among doctors, some maintaining that it was the plague and others denying it. This happened in a great city such as Venice where there are so many and excellent physicians, and from this example I conclude that those indolent sluggards who are always ready to pass judgments on everybody should not marvel at the fact that here in Palermo it took us fifteen or even twenty days to decide whether it was the plague and where it came from.[5]

When the plague epidemic ravaged Northern Italy in 1629, in Milan Dr. Tadino reported that "some physicians kept saying that there was no question of plague";[6] in Bergamo, Dr. Benaglio reported that his colleagues stubbornly maintained "that the disease presently prevailing is not the plague,'"[7] and in Verona, according to Dr. Pona, some physicans "attributed the highly increased mortality to worms," while other maintained that the prevailing fevers "were malignant rather than pestilential.'"[8] Rondinelli, in his report on the epidemic of 1631 in Florence, writes that "physicians were frequently summoned by

---

4. *Merck Manual of Diagnosis and Therapy,* eleventh ed. (1966), p. 850.
5. Ingrassia, *Informatione,* Part 1, pp. 28–30.
6. Tadino, *Raguaglio,* p. 83.
7. Benaglio, "Relazione," pp. 474–78.
8. Pona, *Il gran contagio,* p. 21.

the Health Magistracy, and in these large assemblies they held lengthy discussions on whether it was plague or not. Some physicians maintained that it was the plague, others denied it, and not for the pleasure of contradiction but because they believed so.'"[9]

To explain the apparent paradox of so many doubts and debates when the symptoms of the disease were accurately described, a number of factors must be taken into account. To admit the presence of an epidemic is not an easy step today and was not an easy step in the past. The physician who declared the presence of plague in Busto Arsizio in 1630 was shot to death. Admittedly this was an extreme case, but all physicians who proclaim the presence of a dread disease have to face widespread hostility and unpopularity—to say the least. The psychological importance of social pressures on physicians should not be underrated: men have an extraordinary capacity for self-delusion. However, the role of this factor should not be overestimated either. There were other important elements of an objective nature which stood in the way of a correct diagnosis.

We have learned to distinguish between bubonic and pneumonic plague and some distinguish between bubonic and septicemic plague, though the septicemic form is but the fulminant expression of the bubonic type. Even though the doctors of the sixteenth and seventeenth centuries did not use our terminology, they were aware of the existence of an intriguing variety of conditions, but they could not help being confused and baffled by it. At the end of the sixteenth century Dr. Ingrassia wrote: ''Many physicians mistakenly report that plague is not present when they do not see buboes, anthraxes, papules, spots, or similar signs on the bodies of the deceased.'"[10] The anonymous physician from Bologna whom I quoted above recorded in 1630 that ''at the onset of the epidemic there were doctors who thought it

9. Rondinelli, *Relazione del contagio*, pp. 26–28.
10. Ingrassia, *Informatione*, Part 1, p. 24.

was not the plague if buboes, carbuncles, and splotches did not appear, though later they learned from experience that the plague can be present even without external signs.'"¹¹ Moreover, plague not only presented itself with a variety of symptoms, but many of the symptoms were common to other illnesses, thus making differential diagnosis very difficult, if not altogether impossible. This point, reiterated by a number of writers, was clearly made by Dr. Benaglio when he wrote in 1630:

> Some signs can be said to be typical of the plague, while other signs the plague has in common with other malignant fevers. The signs which are typical are the buboes under the armpit and in the groin and the true carbuncles. The signs which are common to other fevers are the high temperature, the petechiae, the large spots on the skin, parotitis, mental dullness and headache, delirium, sleepiness, vomiting, and cloudy urine. Since these symptoms are common [to a number of diseases] they have frequently been a source of confusion.¹²

Medical writers desperately tried to clarify the whole matter. On the one hand, in an effort to help identification, they lengthened the list of symptoms. At the end of the sixteenth century, Parisi remarked that "among modern writers, Ficino lists fifteen symptoms, Fracastorius nineteen, Fernelius thirty (namely, twelve for ephemeral plague and eighteen for putrefactive plague), Massa twenty-four symptoms in his introduction and fifty-one in chapter six, Fallopius twenty-nine, Ingrassia fifty-two, Mercurialis twenty-six.'"¹³ On the other hand, doctors tried to differentiate among different pathological conditions by multiplying categories, and they made subtle distinctions among "true plague" (*vera pestis*), "pestilential contagion," "pestilential fevers," "ephemeral plague," "putrefactive plague," and the like.¹⁴ The net result was even greater confusion. Quoting Ficino's

11. ASF, Miscellanea Medicea, b. 389.
12. Benaglio, "Relazione," p. 476.
13. Parisi, *Avvertimento*, p. 46.
14. See, for instance, Ingrassia, *Informatione*, Part 2, pp. 95 ff.

Treatise on the Plague, Dr. Parisi commented: "The variety and deceptiveness of the symptoms in the plague and in the pestilential fevers are so great that the physician cannot very easily identify them. If there is one part of medicine which is highly conjectural, it is—to use the Greek name—semeiotics, especially when it deals with the symptoms of plague and of prestilential fevers."[15] In more modern and precise terms, "classification and terminology, which are inseparable, are worthless and may be positively misleading unless built on a sound etiological foundation. To attempt to name and classify pathological conditions on the basis of superficial symptomatic resemblances or speculative notions of pathology is to run the risk of sowing confusion."[16]

When epidemics break out today, clinical examination alone can usually provide the diagnosis, but even today sporadic cases are difficult to diagnose. In such doubtful cases, the modern physician can count on "a sound etiological foundation" and on the concomitant bacteriological confirmation. The current methods of diagnosis are culture and evaluation of smears by fluorescent antibody and, less commonly, the Wayson stain. A few decades ago the pathogen could be identified in the fluid from a bubo (or sputum in the pneumonic type of disease) by culture and guinea pig inoculation. Unfortunately the doctors of the Renaissance did not have the benefit of such tests, and they found themselves in an awkward position, especially when hard pressed by the Health Magistrates to make up their minds.

In most cities of Northern Italy by the end of the sixteenth century, before granting permission to bury the deceased, the health officers requested a death certificate specifying the cause of death. The certificate had to be issued and signed by a certified physician or surgeon. In normal times the routine created no problems and doctors made their diagnoses more or less diligently, according to both their limited knowledge and general

15. Parisi, *Avvertimento*, p. 46.
16. Howard-Jones, "Cholera Nomenclature", p. 323.

fashion or personal taste.[17] But when rumors of plague began to circulate, the health officers became both more demanding and more suspicious. In January 1593 the health officers of Venice became alarmed at a rapidly growing number of cases of illness and deaths on the island of Malamocco. Suspecting the worst, they ordered the exhumation of three bodies that had been buried few days earlier; on the corpses the physician of the Health Magistracy uncovered "at the attachment of the ears" the unmistakable buboes. The island was promptly quarantined.[18]

Exhumations were not an uncommon practice in order to ascertain the cause of death; postmortems before burials were more frequently practiced.[19] The following are two examples of postmortem reports made during the epidemic of 1656–57:[20]

Report on the autopsy of a body made in the pesthouse of the Island [in Rome]: This morning the autopsy of G. G. was performed by me, G. B., surgeon of the Pesthouse of the Island, with the assistance of His Excellency Signor G. B. P., physician of the pesthouse, and of the Rev. Father P., who is also a doctor in this pesthouse.

This is what was found. The exterior part of the body was found to be covered by black petechiae with a black spot as large as a bean in the medial part of the right knee.

Opening the abdomen [we found] the skin to be thick and dry. The muscles of the abdominal wall were of bad color, the fat tissue very dry, the omentum rotten, the guts all black, the peritoneum cyanotic, the stomach very thin, the spleen rotten, the liver doubled in size but of bad color and consistency, the gallbladder full of black bile.

Regarding the thorax, the pleurae were rotten, the pericardium very hard, the mediastinum and the sagittal septum livid, the heart livid

17. For a study of the causes of death as declared by doctors in Milan in the-sixteenth and seventeenth centuries, see Zanetti, "La morte a Milano," pp. 812 ff.

18. ASF, Sanità, Negozi, b. 134, c. 122 (12 January 1593).

19. In 1711 the health board of Venice requested that a number of physicians attend all necropsies of individuals who had died after a short illness. See Archivio di Stato, Venice, Provveditori alla Sanità, b. 80, c. 57 (15 April 1711).

20. The two reports were published by Savio, "Ricerche sulla peste," pp. 139–40.

with its tip black, both ventricles full of very dark blood. The lungs, of bad consistency and color, were all covered with black petechiae.

This is what can be said about the knowledge of this body. 26 October 1656 [signatures follow].

Report on the autopsies of two bodies made in Naples by M. A. S. and F. M.: an autopsy was performed on two bodies, a male and a female, under the instructions of the Illustrious Health Deputies of this city of Naples. The autopsy was performed by the very expert anatomists, M. A. S. and F. M. with the assistance of the Head Physician and other doctors.

It was noticed that all the organs—namely, the heart, lungs, liver, stomach, and guts—were covered with black spots. Moreover, the gallbladder was found full of black bile which was very thick and fattish to the point that it adhered stickily to the inner part of the gallbladder. Especially, however, the major vessels of the heart were full of blood which was clotted and black. This is the summary of the observation.

Knowing how relevant death certificates are to epidemiology and how valuable autopsy data are for a correct assessment of causes of death, we may certainly regard the practice mentioned above as an important step in the history and development of epidemiology. But it must be conceded that the rudimentary technology and the inability to distinguish between pathological and cadaveric conditions made the postmortem reports of the period in question practically useless. Clearly they were of no avail either to the doctors or to the health officers, and only the further spread of an epidemic could bring the arguments among the physicians to an end.

Infectiousness

The doctors and health officers, as well as the educated and semieducated people in general of the Late Middle Ages and Renaissance, largely overestimated the contagiosity of the plague. They exaggerated the possibility that infected objects could transmit the disease to healthy individuals, and in a similar vein they largely overestimated the possibility of interhuman contagion. In the golden age of microbiology, between 1894 and 1908, it was experimentally established that plague is primarily a rat disease, that plague is conveyed from rat to rat by the rat's flea (*Xenopsylla cheopis*), and that fleas are the intermediary ordinarily concerned with the transmission of plague from rat to man. Further research established that direct interhuman contagion occurs solely in the case of pneumonic plague, via droplet infection. Finally, it has been suggested that man → man's flea → man contagion is not a likely event (a) because *Pulex irritans* (the human flea) is not a very efficient vector of *Yersinia pestis* (the pathogen of plague), and (b) because *Yersinia pestis* rarely causes the degree of septicemia in man that it does in the rat, and consequently the flea does not ingest in its meal of human blood a sufficiently large dose of *Yersinia pestis* to enable the bacterium to colonize the flea's stomach. All this is hardly refutable but, strictly interpreted, it may lead to underestimation of the contagiosity of plague in the same way that doctors of the sixteenth and seventeenth centuries overestimated it. In the biological field it is never wise to be dogmatic. Recent research has proven that human fleas and possibly the louse have been capable of transmitting the pathogen from man to man.[21] As to the effectiveness of *Pulex irritans* as a vector, Dr. L. F. Hirst has suggested that in certain environments the human flea possibly compensates in numbers for its intrinsic inferiority to *Xenopsylla cheopis*.[22] The importance of this fact must be viewed in the light of the extremely unsanitary conditions in which people of preindustrial Europe normally lived. Fleas were overly abundant in the dwellings and on the bodies of the rich as well as in the dwellings and on the bodies of the poor. And, of course, fleas were not lacking in the hospitals and pesthouses. Father

21. Baltazard, "Déclin et destin," and Biraben, *Les hommes et la peste*, Vol. 1, pp. 334–35.
22. Hirst, *Conquest of Plague*, pp. 236–46.

Antero writes that fleas were perhaps the worst torment he suffered while serving in the pesthouse at Genoa: they were so numerous and voracious that the poor friar could hardly sleep at night or stand still at the altar while celebrating mass.[23]

Infected fleas (technically called "blocked" fleas) have an ominous capacity to survive from six weeks to up to one year after they have become infected and they can easily lodge in clothes, palliasses, rags, furs, carpets and the like. The suspicion with which the public health officers of the sixteenth and seventeenth centuries regarded the clothes and mattresses of infected people was not absurd.

The health authorities of the time went out of their way to trace the sequence of events which resulted in the spread of infection. The following are only two among the many examples that could be quoted. In the summer of 1631 a laborer from the village of Barberino (where there was no plague) went to Maremma for seasonal work, although that area was infected. Having contracted the disease, the laborer felt the urge to return home, where he died within three days. Fearing the plague, nobody in the village dared approach the body, and his wife and daughter had to bury him. Within a few days one of the two women was dead, and the other was sick, showing the unmistakable bubo.[24] In September 1632 in a house in the suburbs of Florence a man, his son, his daughter, and a nephew died of the plague. Later the man's wife, Sandra Vivoli, also caught the disease. Her son-in-law Simon visited her while she was sick and alone, and within six days he died. A few days later his son and daughter also died. Simon's mother visited him while he was sick, and she too fell prey to the plague.[25] Simon may well have been infected by a blocked rat flea in Sandra Vivoli's house when

23. See above, Chapter 1, footnote 12.
24. ASF, Sanità, Negozi, b. 159, c. 520 (15 July 1631).
25. ASF, Sanità, Negozi, b. 166, c. 634 (15 September 1632).

he visited her and may have carried it home on himself, but it is difficult to believe that the same blocked flea kept jumping from one individual to the next, bringing the plague to three separate households. The case in question seems to support the view of those medical writers who do not reject the possibility of man → human flea → man chain of infection.

Prognosis

Although doctors did not refrain from treating their patients by phlebotomy, emetics, theriacas, vesicants, ointments, and all kinds of other preparations, in general they had little faith in their efforts. Prognosis was poor. As Parisi wrote: "We shall prognosticate death rather than recovery as the disease is malignant, treacherous, pestiferous, and inimical to our vital spirits.[26] As early as the fourteenth and fifteenth centuries, doctors had learned to distinguish between "plague" and "plague with blood spitting"—as witnessed by Guy de Chauliac and Jacopo di Coluccino da Lucca—and those who were alert to the difference were ready to make a more unfavorable prognosis for the pneumonic than for the bubonic form.

Mortality

When statistical information is available about the effects of plague, it generally refers to total mortality. In other words, we are informed about the total number of deaths during an epidemic in the city or area affected by the plague, and if we have some information about the size of the population, we can calculate crude death rates. Quantitative data for periods preceding the sixteenth century must be taken with more than a normal dose of skepticism, but those available for the sixteenth and seventeenth centuries are in general of much better quality. In

26. Parisi, *Avvertimento*, p. 110.

Table A.1. Mortality in Selected Italian Cities during the Epidemics
of 1576–77, 1630–31, 1656–57

Period	City	Population before the epidemic (thousands)	Deaths during the epidemic (thousands)	Deaths as percentage of population
1576–77	Venice	180	50	28%
1630–31	Bergamo	25	10	40
	Bologna	62	15	24
	Brescia	24	11	46
	Carmagnola	7.6	1.9	25
	Como	12	5	42
	Cremona	37	17	46
	Empoli	2.2	0.22	10
	Florence	76	9	12
	Milan	130	60	46
	Modena	18	4	22
	Monza	7	4	57
	Padua	32	19	59
	Parma	30	15	50
	Pescia	2.8	1.4	50
	Pistoia	8	0.12	1.5
	Prato	6	1.5	25
	Venice	140	46	33
	Verona	54	33	61
	Vicenza	32	12	38
1656–57	Genoa	75	45	60
	Naples	300	150	50
	Rome	123	23	19

Table A.1 I have assembled data on population and mortality in selected Italian cities hit by the plague during the three major epidemics of 1576–77, 1630–31, and 1656–57. The list is far from complete because for a number of cities we have no numerical information. As to the data collected, they should not be taken at face value. Statistical accuracy was still in its infancy, and the disruption of urban life caused by an epidemic adversely affected the accuracy of the recording process. Yet the figures in the table can be retained as fairly good indicators of orders of

Table A.2. Mortality in the Rural Communities of the Territory of Empoli (Tuscany) during the Epidemic of 1630–31

Community	Population before the epidemic	Deaths as percentage of population
Cerbaiola	122	—[a]
Corticella e Patignana	70	—
San Bartolomeo	150	—
San Giusto	100	—
Santa Maria	70	—
Vitiana	120	—
San Lorenzo	200	> 0[b]
San Stefano	150	> 0
San Donato	280	2
Pagnano	80	3
Riottoli	50	4
San Giacomo	25	4
Arnovecchio	100	6
Empoli vecchio	150	8
San Andrea e Giovanni	300	8
Cernucchio	118	9
Azzano	170	> 9
Pontorme	340	> 12
Ripa	100	20
Panzano	140	> 47
Cortenuova	370	> 48

Source: Cipolla, "La peste del 1630–31."

[a] Dash indicates that the corresponding locality was free of infection.

[b] Symbol indicates that in addition to the figure given, there were other patients whose destiny was still uncertain at the time of the inquiry.

magnitude: by the end of the sixteenth century Italian cities could boast of a good record of administrative efficiency. The data clearly show that the impact of an epidemic varied greatly, ranging from a crude mortality rate of about 1.5 percent in one city to about 61 percent in another—with by far the great majority of cases falling between 21 and 50 percent. In other words, when an epidemic of plague broke out in a community the chances were that from one-quarter to one-half of the population would disappear unpleasantly in a matter of few months.

One has no difficulty in understanding the terror that the mere mention of the plague inspired among the people of the time.

When the plague hit an urban center, most of those who could afford it left the town for the countryside. This fact has led some historians to believe that plague epidemics were mostly urban affairs. The available evidence, however, does not corroborate this view. When an epidemic of plague flared up in a given area, some rural communities escaped the infection but many did not, and in the affected villages the demographic losses produced by the plague were proportionately as great as in the towns.[27] During the epidemic of 1630–31 an officer of the Health Magistracy in Florence produced a valuable report on the effects of the plague in the territory of Empoli (see Fig. 7, p. 52). The basic data of the report are assembled in Table A.2. They show that out of 21 rural communities ranging in size from 25 to 370 souls and with a total population of 3,205 people, 6 localities with 632 inhabitants, namely 29 percent of the communities accounting for 20 percent of the population, escaped the infection. The other communities as a whole lost together about 25 percent of their population. As in the cases of the major cities, the mortality rates for individual communities varied noticeably, ranging from 2 and 3 percent in the cases of San Donato and Pagnano and possibly less in the cases of San Giusto and San Stefano to more than 47 and more than 48 percent in the cases of Panzano and Cortenuova.[28] Since the fatality rate in the case of bubonic plague varies within relatively narrow limits, the wide dispersion of mortality rates both in the cities and the

27. See also the observations by Gottfried, *Epidemic Disease in Fifteenth-Century England*, pp. 138 ff., 226.

28. See Cipolla, "La peste del 1630–31." Similar conclusions have been reached by Billiet ("Notice sur la peste"), who studied the epidemic of 1630 in the diocese of Maurienne in Savoy. In 55 rural communities, mortality ranged from 1 percent in one community to 48 percent in another. See also Biraben, *Les hommes et la peste*, Vol. 1, p. 228.

rural communities suggests noticeable differences in the incidence of morbidity from one place to another.

It has been asserted that ''the less time the plague lasted, the higher the total proportion that died.''[29] Phrased in this way, the statement sounds paradoxical. In fact, all that is meant is that if a plague epidemic was particularly intense and lethal it could not last long. Even if expressed in this more sensible way, however, the proposition cannot be left unargued as it may falsely suggest a functional relationship between duration and severity. Biological phenomena, especially when compounded with social complexities, are never so simply definable. There have been cases of short epidemics with high total mortality, there have been cases of short epidemics with low total mortality, and there have been cases of long epidemics with high mortality.[30]

Morbidity and Case Fatality

In his *Observations*, the Swiss physician Felix Platter reported that during the plague epidemic which struck Basel at the beginning of 1610 and lasted until the end of March of the following year, 6,408 persons became infected and 3,968 died.[31] Before

29. Hollingsworth, *Historical Demography*, pp. 365 ff.

30. Epidemics are very complex phenomena, and superficial comparison among epidemics which are distant in time and space is a risky proposition. If, however, we compare in Table A.1 two epidemics which took place at practically the same time (1630–31) in two cities—Prato and Pistoia—less than 20 miles apart and with similar cultural, economic, and social structures, we find that the epidemic lasted longer in Prato than in Pistoia and killed more people in Prato (some 25 percent of the population) than in Pistoia (about 1.5 percent of the population). This example contradicts the hypothesis by Hollingsworth mentioned above in the text.

If one compares the epidemic which afflicted Milan and Pistoia one finds a similarity of timing and yet an extraordinary dissimilarity in mortality.

31. Platter, *Observationum*, pp. 321–22. According to Bickel ("Über die Pest in der Schweiz," pp. 513 ff.), Platter's figures should be adjusted to exclude those who died for reasons other than the plague. He suggests the figures of 3600 deaths due to the plague over approximately 6000 infected. This correction does not affect the percentages calculated in the text above.

Table A.3. Infection and Mortality in Four Tuscan Communities, 1631

Community	Duration of epidemic	Initial population	Number infected	Deaths
San Gimignano	18 February– 2 October 1631	2,000	962	670
Sasso	4 October 1631– 2 January 1632	190	100	60
Castel Val Cecina	20 July– 16 November 1631	485	185	121
Cozzile	16 July– 9 October 1631	280	225	141

Source: ASF, Sanità, Negozi, b. 161, c. 849; b. 162, c. 521; b. 164, cc. 149 and 191. For Cozzile, see also AS Pescia, Archivio Comunale, b. 193, c. 329.

Table A.4. Rates of Mobidity, Case Fatality, and Mortality
in the Same Four Tuscan Communities (*percentages*)

Community	Morbidity	Case fatality	Mortality
San Gimignano	48	70	33
Sasso	52	60	32
Castel Val Cecina	38	65	25
Cozzile	80	63	50

the epidemic, the population of Basel was approximately 15,000 inhabitants. We can therefore roughly estimate the following rates: *morbidity* (number infected over total population) = 43 percent; *case fatality* (number of deaths over number infected) = 62 percent; *mortality* (number of deaths over total population) = 26 percent. In other words, almost half of the population contracted the disease, the case fatality rate was about 60 percent, and consequently, more than one-quarter of the population of the city died during the fifteen-month epidemic.

About seventy years after Platter wrote his *Observations*, a plague epidemic struck Tuscany. The reports of the local health commissioners for four small Tuscan communities provide the data given in Table A.3. The rates derived from those data are given in Table A.4.

Table A.5. Case Fatality Rates during Limited Periods of Epidemics
in Three Tuscan Communities, 1631

Community	Period	Number infected	Deaths	Case fatality (percent)
Colle	4–30 August 1631	61	37	61
Pratovecchio	24 September–31 December 1631	68	48	71
Empoli	24 June–15 July 1631	37	16	43

Sources: For Colle, AFS, Sanità, Negozi, b. 160, c. 907 (30 August 1631); for Pratovecchio, ibid., b. 164, c. 195 (no date); for Empoli, ibid., b. 159, cc. 582 ff. (17 July 1631).

In these four cases, the morbidity rate varied from more than one-third to 80 percent of the population and the case fatality rate varied from 60 to 70 percent.

In addition to these four communities, other communities were covered in the reports of the Tuscan health commissioners during the epidemic of 1631, but those reports do not allow the assessment of morbidity and total mortality. Either they fail to provide information on the size of the total population at risk, or they refer only to a limited period of the epidemic. For the period covered, however, they allow calculation of fatality rates, shown in Table A.5.

In summary, the Tuscan evidence relating to the epidemic of 1630–31 suggests fatality rates ranging from 60 to 71 percent in six communities out of seven and at 43 percent in the seventh. The results are consistent with those reached by historians who studied epidemics of plague in other parts of Europe during the sixteenth and seventeenth centuries and who observed fatality rates ranging from 47 to 78 percent.[32] The results are also con-

32. The average fatality rate stood at 77 percent at Apt (France) in 1588, 47 percent at Igualada (Spain) in 1589, 59 percent at Basel (Switzerland) in 1610–11, 71 percent at Dunkerque (France) in 1666, 65 percent at Gravelines (France) in 1666, 78 percent in Provence in 1720–22. See Platter, *Observationum,* pp. 321–22; Biraben, *Les hommes et la peste,* p. 303; Revel, "Autour d'une épidémie," p. 970.

sistent with observations made by modern epidemiologists in the plague epidemics of the nineteenth and twentieth centuries in India and Manchuria: in these instances it was observed that fatality rates for the bubonic form ranged from 60 to 80 percent.[33]

Differential Morbidity and Differential Mortality

At the time, practically everybody agreed that the incidence of plague was much greater among the lower orders than among the upper classes, and if one considers the overcrowded and unsanitary conditions in which the mass of the working population lived, one has no difficulty in accepting this view.[34] Whether the fatality rate varied among different social classes, and if so, how it varied, was—and still is—a debatable question. Dr. Ingrassia thought that both morbidity and fatality were higher among the poor. Dr. Parisi thought that morbidity was higher among the poor ''because of the misery and distress in which they always live,'' but that fatality was higher among the upper classes because ''the nobility is more delicate and tender and less strong.'' Both doctors based their opinions on haphazard observation, guess, and speculation, and neither substantiated his opinion with facts. Father Antero, superintendent of the pesthouse at Genoa during the epidemic of 1656–57, shared Parisi's view when he concluded that ''the privilege of the rich consists of their being able to avoid the plague while the privilege of the poor consists in the fact that they can survive the plague when they catch it.''[35]

The average fatality rate did not remain constant during an epidemic. While recognizing this fact, Shrewsbury maintained that ''in most of the European epidemics of bubonic plague from

33. Pollitzer, *Plague*, p. 418; Wu, *Manchurian Plague*, p. 82; Simpson, *Treatise*, p. 313.

34. Biraben, "Les pauvres et la peste," pp. 506–7; Cipolla and Zanetti, "Peste et mortalité," pp. 197–202.

35. See Cipolla, "Plague and the Malthusians," pp. 280–83.

the fourteenth to the end of the seventeenth century, the case fatality rate appears to have approached 90 percent in the initial weeks of an epidemic, though it commonly fell as low as 30 percent as the epidemic subsided.[36] That proposition is untenable. According to Dr. Ingrassia, during the epidemic which struck Palermo (Sicily) in 1575, "At the beginning the greatest part of the patients recovered," while later on "the disease became more cruel day by day."[37] Canon Cini, a clergyman who was also a physician, noticed the same phenomenon in Poggibonsi (Tuscany) during the epidemic of 1632-33: "While earlier some of those who became sick recovered, now all die and in very short time."[38] Father Antero had a similar experience in the pesthouse of Genoa during the epidemic of 1656-57. The pesthouse was opened on September 13, 1656, and, according to Father Antero, "During the first months no less than one-third of the patients survived . . . by the beginning of the following July only four percent survived."[39] On the other hand, in other places events allegedly run a totally different course, conforming to the pattern hypothesized by Dr. Shrewsbury. According to Dr. Benaglio, during the epidemic of 1630 in Bergamo, "At the beginning the disease was more malignant and few recovered."[40] In Bologna, again during the epidemic of 1630, according to a local physician, "At the beginning and the height of this dreadful scourge very few infected survived. Then, by the beginning of July it seemed as if the sharp ferocity of [death's] scythe lost something of its edge, though very many still died."[41] Thus the available evidence suggests that in some epidemics the fatality rate was on average higher in the early phases of the tragedy than in the later phases, whereas in other

36. Shrewsbury, *History*, p. 5.
37. Ingrassia, *Informatione*, Part 1, p. 70.
38. ASF, Sanità, Negozi, b. 168, c. 783 (10 May 1633).
39. Antero, *Li lazaretti*, pp. 9, 10, 23.
40. Benaglio, "Relazione," p. 464.
41. ASF, Miscellanea Medicea, b. 389.

epidemics the reverse was true. Actually, curious discrepancies could also be observed from one week to the next. In the city of Empoli (Tuscany) from June 21 to 28, 1631, out of 12 new cases only one proved fatal, thus producing a fatality rate of 8 percent. During the following week 34 new cases occurred and 19 were fatal, a fatality rate of 56 percent.[42] Admittedly the number of cases involved is very small and, moreover, there is no possibility of controlling the validity of the diagnosis and other concomitant circumstances; nevertheless, the data in question clearly suggest that one has to be cautious about generalizations.

The Course of Illness

The people of the later Middle Ages and the Renaissance were perfectly aware that once clinical manifestations of the disease had appeared, the disease ran a rapid course, and that in fatal cases it unfailingly proved to be a fast killer. Montaigne maintained that death from plague was not one of the worst because "it is usually quick."[43] Listing the elements on the basis of which doctor could pronounce plague as a cause of death, Dr. Ingrassia put "primarily instant death or death which occurs within two, three, or four days at the most."[44] The anonymous physician who reported on the epidemic of 1630 in Bologna noted that "some died within one day, some in a matter of one hour, some in the fourth day, some in the seventh, and some also later."[45] In Florence, Rondinelli reported that "death ordinarily occurred by the seventh day, and for some it occurred by the fourth."[46] When the documents allow us to study the stories of individual cases, we find further confirmation that the disease

---

42. ASF, Sanità, Negozi, b. 159, cc. 582 ff. (17 July 1631).
43. Montaigne, *Essays*, III, 12.
44. Ingrassia, *Informatione*, Part 1, p. 106.
45. ASF, Miscellanea Medicea, b. 389.
46. Rondinelli, *Relazione del contagio*, p. 31.

unfailingly followed a rapid course and death, when it occurred, resulted in a few days.[47]

The Course of Epidemics

Epidemics of plague could randomly start in the spring months, in the summer, or in the fall. If an epidemic broke out late in the year it might spread in the winter months. The minuscule village of San Piero Grignano (near Florence) was literally devastated by the plague during the fall of 1630 and the winter of 1631, as shown by the following figures:[48]

Month	Deaths
September 1630	2
October	0
November	15
December	22
January 1631	14
February	16
March	13

The case of San Piero Grignano was, however, exceptional. As a rule an epidemic of plague subsided during the cold months of January and February.

47. As an example among many I quote here the notation entered by a terrorized priest in the book of the deceased of the parish of San Matteo of Pistoia (Archivio Vescovile, Pistoia) on November 20, 1630: "On Sunday the 17th, while attending mass in San Matteo, Signora Margherita, daughter of Signor Francesco Dazzi, General Secretary of this City, almost fainted and thus went home to bed where it was found that she had a malignant fever with pain in the thigh. She was visited by surgeons who applied anointed woolens and oil of white lilies. On Wednesday morning she was visited again by Master Pietro Segni, surgeon of this City. A suction cup was applied to her thigh where there was a small tumor. This was incised twice and then drawing ointments were applied. But two hours and one half after dusk of the same day she passed from this life to Heaven and in fact some say that she died, Ave Maria, of plague. I priest Domenico Giustini, unworthy confessor of the Signora, gave to her the Holy Sacraments and, thanks to God, I managed to escape and for this I must highly praise God, the always glorious virgin Mary, San Domenico, and all Saints, both male and female, who are my protectors and also I must be thankful forever to the Most Holy Trinity."

48. ASF, Sanità, Negozi, b. 156, c. 79 (27 March 1631).

The curve of a plague epidemic roughly conforms to a bell-shaped pattern, but it can be skewed to the right or to the left. The various degrees of distortion from symmetry remind us that to a large extent every outbreak is a unique historical event. Occasionally one encounters a two-wave curve (see for example Fig. 8, above, p. 60). The trough of such a curve also normally coincides with the winter months.

All this fits what we know about the etiology of the plague. The advent of frosty weather in winter causes a lowering of the rat-flea density because the fleas either hibernate or die and the rats seemingly calm down in their sexual activity. With a low rat-flea density an epidemic is likely to die out. If, however, *Yersinia pestis* is kept viable and virulent by an enzootic of rat-plague in colonies of house-rats throughout the winter, a recrudescence of epizootic and epidemic plague may occur in the ensuing spring.

Historical evidence and modern scientific knowledge thus confirm the view which was prevalent in the Renaissance—namely, that warm weather greatly favored the spread of the contagion while cold winter weather generally acted as a deterrent.

Agreement Reached between the Grand Duchy of Tuscany and the Republic of Genoa, 1652

On September 5, 1652, replying to a specific request from the Health Magistracy in Florence, the Health Magistracy of Genoa sent a letter enclosing a memorandum of public health procedures followed in the port of Genoa. The Florentine magistrates then requested similar information from the Health Magistracy of Leghorn and forwarded this information to Genoa on September 17. The document below[1] reproduces the text (G) transmitted from Genoa to Florence, and the reply (L) on each separate count that Florence sent to Genoa concerning the corresponding practices in Leghorn.

1. (G) All vessels coming from Catalonia, the islands of Sardinia, Majorca, and Minorca, the province of Languedoc—cities and places banned because of contagion—usually observe complete quarantine, and if there are goods in these ships not subject to contagion their unloading is allowed under supervision of some health officers, every precaution being taken so that people on land have no dealings with those on board.

(L) Agrees with this.

---

1. The document is preserved in ASF, Sanità, Negozi, b. 187, cc. 778 ff. (17 September 1652) and ASF, Mediceo, b. 2327. See also ASF, Sanità, Partiti, b. 13, c. 26 (10 September 1652).

2. (G) If perchance any deaths occur in said vessels, or if anyone falls sick during the voyage or during the time the quarantine is being observed, the quarantine is to be extended for 50 or 60 days according to the danger and circumstances; the people and the goods are to be sent to the pesthouse, including the ship's sails and tackle, while guards on land watch the ships, although it seems that wood does not suffer contagion.

(L) Agrees and is even more rigorous when need requires it.

3. (G) But now that there are so many infected cities, provinces, islands, and places, vessels carrying woolen cloth and other things subject to contagion are not admitted, but are turned back, as happened recently to two that arrived with cloth from Catalonia; even though they belonged to our citizens and the business concerned this market place, they were turned back with threats of pain of death and the burning of their ships if they stayed, and the owners were even obliged to give security that they would not touch any port in the dominion of the Most Serene Republic.

(L) Agrees with this; the same is done at Leghorn also.

4. (G) Vessels coming from parts uninfected but under suspicion are subject to quarantine for 30 or 35 days according to the suspicion held, but nevertheless the goods are sent immediately to the pesthouse.

(L) The same is done at Leghorn.

5. (G) Vessels coming from Cagliari in Sardinia with goods not subject to contagion are to observe 40 days quarantine, and before they only had to do 30 or 35. This is practiced even if notice has been received that people in Cagliari are healthy, as in any case there is danger during the passage, through the dealings they may have with ships and particularly those coming from the said island of Sardinia.

(L) The Health Magistracy at Leghorn has acted and acts in the same way.

6. (G) Foodstuffs are accepted with caution, and cheeses are flooded with sea water so that they are thoroughly washed off, and also the wrappings that are around them, even if made of grass. Cheeses from Majorca are accepted when washed off in vinegar, as the above method is not followed because they would suffer too much.

(L) Although this is not censured, it is not done in Leghorn, nor are cheeses admitted under any circumstances.

7. (G) Vessels from the Levant are quarantined for 30, 35, 40 days according to information received and if they come with a clean bill; the goods at the pesthouse are purified for the same length of time. Purification starts from the day all bales, etc. are opened.

(L) For vessels from the Levant with clean bills it is usual at Leghorn to give permission to land to the Captain and clerk immediately on arrival and to send the goods to the pesthouse. After three days permission is given to the passengers, and the goods have to undergo 15 to 20 days of airing at the pesthouse.

For vessels with unclean bills of health the usual rigorous quarantine.

8. (G) Vessels from England, if they come directly without touching at infected or suspected places, and with clean bills, are allowed entry after a few days; first, however, goods and merchandise are sent to the pesthouse where they are purified for 20 days, and if they touch any of the above [infected] places they must observe complete quarantine.

(L) Agree; the same is done at Leghorn; entry, however, is granted to the Captain and clerk.

9. (G) The same is set down for vessels from Flanders. It is, however, true that purification for merchandise is only 15 days.

(L) The same is observed at Leghorn.

10. (G) Goods coming from Provence that derive from the Levant and other infected places like Languedoc, even though they have bills issued in Provence, are sent to the pesthouse for 15 days' purification; and this is for greater caution, because it has been observed that the bales from the Levant with the Levantine bindings, easily recognized by experienced persons, sometimes come from Provence with clean bills.

(L) This is practiced for [people and merchandise coming from] all places in Provence because they do not have pesthouses. Marseilles, however, has a pesthouse where they now air out the merchandise as is done in Leghorn and Genoa; [therefore, regarding the merchandise proceeding from Marseilles] when accompanied by bills, if it comes from the Levant it is admitted, but the woolen serge from Languedoc, because of a suspicion that it had not been opened and aired but only quarantined in the pesthouse, is sent to the pesthouse for quarantine.

When the signs are recognized, the same care will be taken at Leghorn.

11. (G) Vessels coming from Spain and Ibiza have in the past done 25 days of quarantine. In the future the quarantine will be regulated according to information received, bearing in mind that they maintain trade with Barcelona, where the army is infected, and that the latest news from Ibiza is that great mortality had ensued.

(L) The same will be done at Leghorn too.

With reference to the preceding text, in their communication to Genoa of September 17, 1652, the Health Magistrates of Florence made the following comments:

it seems to us that there is agreement in all the important sections, and in the others the differences do not seem to be of such a nature that needs to be taken into account; therefore we do not doubt that your Lordships will approve that we proceed with this agreement, assuring you that at Leghorn it will be observed with due punctuality, and so long as we do not hear from you to the contrary we shall undertake to have assurances that the same or similar diligence is used in Rome and Naples.

Three days later, on September 20, Genoa replied:[2]

we see from the replies that we agree except in the reception of cheeses, but as you see from the method followed caution is exercised. In respect to vessels coming from the Levant, we too, when they come with a clean bill, shall not fail to grant entry to the Captain and clerk, making them change clothes, and after a certain time entry will also be given to passengers, but before the ship's hold is opened. As far as concerns the merchandise that comes from the Levant via Provence, because bales of merchandise are frequently sent here with bills stating that they have been purified, but are seen here to have the same packaging as from the Levant—well recognized here—because of this they they are sent to the pesthouse for purification.

On our part, therefore, we shall continue the usual practice in order to proceed in concert.

On October 1 the Florentine authorities acknowledged receipt of the Genoese letter of September 20, and in connection with the few points still unsettled they pointed out:[3]

Inasmuch as you have written to us about the cheeses from Sardinia and Majorca, we have nothing further to say except that Leghorn will continue to act as already indicated to you, i.e., not receiving any from either of the above regions. Concerning the merchandise arriving from the Levant that comes via Provence, the same rules will be applied at Leghorn as those which your Lordships cause to be applied at Genoa, and thus we shall proceed harmoniously in all points.

2. ASF, Mediceo, b. 2327.
3. ASF, Mediceo, b. 2327.

Bibliography

Abrate, M. *Popolazione e peste del 1630 a Carmagnola.* Turin, 1973.

Antero, M. da San Bonaventura [F. Micone]. *Li lazaretti della città e riviere di Genova del 1657.* Genoa, 1658.

Baltazard, M. "Déclin et destin d'une maladie infectieuse, la peste." *Bulletin de l'Organisation Mondiale de la Santé* 23 (1960).

Battistini, M. *Le epidemie in Volterra dal 1004 al 1880.* Volterra, 1916.

Beloch, K. J. *Bevölkerungsgeschichte Italiens.* Berlin, 1930–61.

Benaglio, M. A. "Relazione della carestia e della peste di Bergamo e suo territorio negli anni 1629 e 1630." *Miscellanea di Storia Italiana* 6 (1865).

Bernardino, Tomitano. *Consiglio sopra la peste di Venezia l'anno 1556.* Padua, 1556.

Bickel, W. "Uber die Pest in der Schweiz." *Studium Generale* 9 (1956).

Billiet. "Notice sur la peste qui a affligé la diocèse de Maurienne en 1630." *Mémoire de l'Académie de Savoie* 8 (1857).

Bini, M. "La peste dell'anno 1631." *Bollettino Storico Empolese* 5 (1961–62).

Biraben, J. N. *Les hommes et la peste en France et dans les pays européens et méditerranéens.* 2 vols. Paris, 1975.

Biraben, J. N. "Les pauvres et la peste." *Etudes sur l'histoire de la pauvreté,* ed. E. Mollat. Paris, 1974.

Borelli, G. B. *Editti antichi e nuovi.* Turin, 1681.

Brighetti, A. *Bologna e la peste del 1630.* Bologna, 1968.

Burnet, F. M., and White, D. O. *Natural History of Infectious Diseases.* Cambridge, 1972.

Catellacci, D., ed. "Curiosi ricordi del contagio di Firenze del 1630." *Archivio Storico Italiano,* Ser. 5, Vol. 20 (1897).

Ciano, C., *La Sanità Marittima nell'età medicea.* Pisa, 1976.

Cipolla, C. M. *Cristofano and the Plague: A Study in the History of Public Health in the Age of Galileo.* London, Berkeley, 1973.

Cipolla, C. M. *Faith, Reason, and the Plague in Seventeenth-Century Tuscany.* Brighton, Eng., Ithaca, N.Y., 1979.

Cipolla, C. M. "La peste del 1630–31 nell'Empolese." *Archivio Storico Italiano.* 1978.

Cipolla, C. M. "The Plague and the pre-Malthus Malthusians." *The Journal of European Economic History* 3 (1974).

Cipolla, C. M. *Public Health and the Medical Profession in the Renaissance.* Cambridge, 1976.

Cipolla, C. M., and Zanetti, D. E. "Peste et mortalité differentielle." *Annales de Démographie Historique* (1972).

Consoli Fiego, G. *Peste e carestie in Pistoia.* Pistoia, 1920.

Contardo, G. A. *Il modo di preservarsi e curarsi dalla peste.* Genoa, 1576.

Corradi, A. *Annali delle epidemie occorse in Italia dalle prime memorie fino al 1850.* Bologna, 1867–92.

Costa, A. "La peste in Genova negli anni 1656–7." *Atti del Convegno Internazionale per gli studi sulla popolazione.* Vol. 1. Rome, 1933.

Del Panta, L. *Una traccia di storia demografica della Toscana nei secoli XVI–XVIII.* Florence, 1974.

Ferrari, C. *L'Ufficio della Sanità di Padova.* Venice, 1909.

Gastaldi, H. *Tractatus de avertenda et profliganda peste.* Bologna, 1684.

Giuffré, L. "L'epidemia d'influenza del 1557 in Palermo e le proposte per il risanamento della città fatte nel 1558." *Archivio Storico Siciliano,* New Ser. 15 (1890).

Gottfried, R. S. *Epidemic Disease in Fifteenth-Century England: The Medical Response and the Demographic Consequences.* New Brunswick, N.J. 1978.

Hirst, L. F. *The Conquest of Plague.* Oxford, 1953.

Hollingsworth, T. H. *Historical Demography.* London, 1969.

Howard-Jones, N. "Choleranomalies: The Unhistory of Medicine as Exemplified by Cholera." *Perspectives in Biology and Medicine,* 1972.

Howard-Jones, N. "Cholera Nomenclature and Nosology: A Historical Note." *Bulletin of the World Health Organization* 51 (1974).

Howard-Jones, N. *The Scientific Background of the International Sanitary Conferences, 1851–1938.* Geneva, 1975.

Ingrassia, G. F. *Informatione del pestifero e contagioso morbo il quale affligge et have afflitto questa città di Palermo.* Palermo, 1576.

Ingrassia, G. F. *Ragionamento fatto alla presenza del Magistrato sopra le infermità epidemiali e popolari successi nell'anno 1558.* Palermo, 1560.

Manger. *Traité de la peste.* Geneva, 1721.

Parenti, G. *Prime ricerche sulla rivoluzione dei prezzi in Firenze.* Florence, 1939.

Parisi, P. *Avvertimento sopra la peste e febre pestifera.* Palermo, 1593.

Pellegrini, F. *Per la storia della lotta contro le epidemie: sui provvedimenti di profilassi presi dall'Ufficio di Sanità di Verona durante le epidemie del 1575 e 1576.* Verona, 1932.

Pellicini, A. *Discorso sopra de mali contagiosi.* Florence, 1630.

Piattoli, R. *Guida storica e bibliografica degli archivi e delle biblioteche d'Italia.* Rome, 1932.

Platter, F. *Observationum in hominibus affectibus plerisque corpori et animo functionum laesione dolore aliave molestia et vitio incommodantibus, libri tres.* Basel, 1680.

Pollitzer, R. *The Plague.* Geneva, 1954.

Pona, F. *Il gran contagio di Verona nel 1630.* Verona, 1631.

Pullan, B. *Rich and Poor in Renaissance Venice.* Oxford, 1971.

Revel, J. "Autour d'une épidémie ancienne: la peste de 1666–1670." *Revue d'Histoire Moderne et Contemporaine* 17 (1970).

Rondinelli, F. *Relazione del contagio stato in Firenze l'anno 1630 e 1633.* Florence, 1634.

Salvi, M. *Delle historie di Pistoia e fazioni d'Italia.* Venice, 1662.

Salzmann, C. "Masques portés par les médecins en temps de peste." *Aesculape* 22 (1932).

Savio, P. "Ricerche sulla peste di Roma degli anni 1656–1657." *Archivio della Società Romana di Storia Patria* 95 (1972).

Shrewsbury, J. F. D. *A History of Bubonic Plague in the British Isles.* Cambridge, 1970.

Simpson, W. J. *A Treatise on Plague.* Cambridge, 1905.

Tadino, A. *Raguaglio dell'origine et giornali successi della gran peste.* Milan, 1684.

Thomas, L. *The Lives of a Cell: Notes of a Biology Watcher.* New York, 1974.

Toniolo Fascione, M. C. "L'attività processuale del Magistrato di Sanità di Livorno tra il 1650 e il 1659." *Studi Storici e Geografici* 1 (1977).

Wu, Lien-Teh, ed., *Manchurian Plague Prevention Service.* Shanghai, 1934.

Zanetti, D. E. "La morte a Milano." *Rivista Storica Italiana* 88 (1976).

Index

Mattresses: burning of, 15–17, 98
Medici, Cardinal Giovan Carlo de',
    11n7
Medici, Ferdinand II de's, Grand
    Duke of Tuscany, 23–26, 28, 31,
    33, 34, 45, 56–57
Mercurialis, 93
Miasmas: as cause of plague, 8, 12,
    14, 15, 53, 72, 74, 81
Milan, 5, 21, 30, 31, 45; death rate in
    hospitals, 42n36
Modena, 21, 30, 31, 45
Montaigne, Michel Eyquem de, 108
Monte Lupo, 51, 54
Monti, Dr.: in mission to Genoa,
    34–35, 39–42, 44
Mortality. See Plague

Naples: public health system, 5, 49;
    in proposed convention on public
    health, 48, 49
Nencini, Nofri, *Provveditore* of
    Pistoia, 56, 58n

Pagnano, 102
Palermo: plague epidemic of 1575,
    107
Palliasses: burning of, 15–17, 98
Panzano, 102
Parisi, Dr. P., 93–94, 99, 106
Parma, 15, 21, 23, 30, 45
Pellicini, Dr. Antonio, 89–90
Pesthouses: fleas in, 12, 12–13n12,
    97–98; Genoa, 12, 38–40, 98;
    Pistoia, 55, 58–66, 68, 70–71,
    75–77
Piacenza, 15
Pianosa: suspended, 27, 28, 30, 31
Piombino: suspended, 27, 28, 30, 31
Pisa: health board, 24; plague control
    in, 24, 25; plague epidemic of
    1630–31, 51
Pistoia: plague epidemic of 1630–31,
    51–85, 103n30; Health Deputies,
    52–57, 59, 61, 62–63, 65, 66, 68,
    69, 71, 75, 76, 80, 81, 84; clean-

liness enforced, 52, 53–54; silkworms prohibited, 53; foreigners,
mountebanks, and Jews expelled,
53, 83; surgeons and barbers as
sources of infection, 54; trade with
Florence temporarily forbidden, 54;
public health expenditures, 55, 66–
75; pesthouses (lazaretti), 55, 58–
66, 68, 70–71, 75–81; clergy op-
pose public health measures, 56;
mortality rate in plague, 58, 65–66,
78–85; charity as source of reve-
nue, 66–68; food expenditures by
Health Deputies, 68–70; convalescent homes, 68, 71–72; wages of
health service personnel, 70–71;
burial of plague victims, 72–73,
81–82; quarantine of poor and
well-to-do patients, 76–79; houses
of plague victims locked, 77–79;
typhus epidemic of 1628–29, 83,
84–85; population affected by
plague, 83–84
Plague: pandemic of 1348, 3; epidemic of 1576, 7; causes of, in early
theories, 8, 13–15; epidemic of
1630–31, 23, 51, 91, 92, 104–5,
107, 108, 109. (*See also* Pistoia);
mortality and fatality rates in
Pistoia, 58, 65–66, 78–85; early
treatment of, 64, 99; burial of victims, 72–73, 81–82; in U.S., cases
caused by animals, 74n47; symptoms and signs, 89–91; diagnosis, 91–96; bubonic, pneumonic,
distinguished, 92–94; death certificates, 94–95, 96; postmortems,
95–96; infectiousness, 96–99;
prognosis, 99; mortality, total, 99–
103; morbidity and case fatality,
103–6; differential morbidity and
differential mortality, 106–8;
course of illness, 108–9; course of
epidemics, seasonal effects, 109–10
Plague control, 3–5, 7, 8; cleaning of
environment, 15–16, 52, 53–54;

Plague control (continued)
interstate relations, 19–50; clothing
of victims, 72; personal belongings
of victims, 73. *See also* Quarantine
Platter, Felix, 103
Pneumonic plague, 92, 97, 99
Poggibonsi: plague epidemic of
1632–33, 107
Pona, Dr. F., 11n6, 91
Postmortems, 95–96
Poverty, 3, 73; poor patients in
hospitals and pesthouses, 76–77;
morbidity and fatality rates of
plague among poor, 106
Prato: plague in, 51, 55, 71n42,
73n46, 79, 84, 103n30
Pratovecchio, 105
Prescia, Giovanni, 12n9
Public health systems: Northern Italy,
3–4; outside of Italy, 4
Pulex irritans, 97
Pullan, Brian, 67

Quarantine: in Florence, 17–18; in
Leghorn, 32; in Genoa pesthouse,
39; in Pistoia, of poor and well-to-
do patients, 76–77; houses locked,
77–79

Rats, 14, 75, 85, 97, 110
Rickettsia prowaceki, 85
Robe of waxed cloth, 9–14, 17
Rome: public health system, 5; doctor's robe in, 12; Tuscany banished
by, 25; Genoa and Corsica suspended by, 30–31; in proposed
convention on public health, 34,
43, 48–49; plague epidemic of
1656–57; 90
Rondinelli, Dr. F., 15, 91–92, 108
Rosetta, 31

San Donato, 102
San Gimignano, 104
San Giusto, 102
San Piero Grignano, 109
San Stefano, 102

Sardinia: suspended, 19–21; plague
in, 23, 24, 26–27; banished, 25;
boats from, in Genoa, 26–27, 30
Sasso, 104
Scotti, Monsignor, 48
Septicemic plague, 92
Shrewsbury, Dr. J. F. D., 106–7
Sicily: influenza epidemic of 1557, 7
Siena: *Balía*, 4
Silkworms: prohibited, 53
Silvestri, Signor: in mission to Genoa,
34–37, 39, 42–45
Spinola, Giovanni Antonio, 43, 45
Suspension: banishment distinguished
from, 19, 21

Tadino, Dr. A., 91
Tavola, 51
Trespiano, 51
Tuscany, Grand Duchy of: Supreme
Health Magistracy, 23–24, 52;
plague control in relations with
Genoa, 24–27, 28, 30, 31, 32; banished by Rome, 25; convention on
public health proposed by, 34, 43,
46–50; suspension of Genoa repealed, 45–46; agreement with
Genoa (1652), 46–50 (text, 111–
15); plague epidemic of 1630–31,
51, 104–5, 109
Tuscany, Grand Duke of. *See* Medici,
Ferdinand II de'
Typhus: epidemic of 1648, 25;
epidemic in Genoa, 1649, 33n32;
epidemic in Pistoia, 1628–29, 83,
84–85

Venice, Republic of, 5, 21, 30, 45;
plague in, 95
Verona, 21, 30
Vettori, Luigi, Marquis: report on
plague in Pistoia, 57–59, 65, 66,
75, 76–78, 80–84

Xenopsylla cheopis, 97

Yersinia pestis, 3, 74n41, 85, 97, 110

DESIGNED BY IRVING PERKINS ASSOCIATES
COMPOSED BY FOX VALLEY TYPESETTING
MENASHA, WISCONSIN
MANUFACTURED BY MALLOY LITHOGRAPHING, INC.
ANN ARBOR, MICHIGAN
TEXT IS SET IN HOLLAND SEMINAR AND SABON
DISPLAY LINES ARE SET IN HOLLAND SEMINAR

Library of Congress Cataloging in Publication Data
Cipolla, Carlo M
Fighting the plague in seventeenth-century Italy.
(The Curti lectures; 1978)
Bibliography: pp. 117–19
Includes index.
1. Plague—Italy—History. I. Title.
II. Series: Merle Curti lectures; 1978.
[DNLM: 1. Plague—History—Italy. 2. History of medicine,
17th century—Italy. WC 350 C577fa]
RC178.I8C56   614.5′732′0945   80-5111
ISBN 0-299-08340-3
ISBN 0-299-08344-6 (pbk.)